The Elixir of Platelet Rich Plasma Therapy in Intervention Dermatology and Regenerative Trichology

The Elixir of Platelet Rich Plasma Therapy in Intervention Dermatology and Regenerative Trichology

Edited by

Suruchi Garg

Cambridge Scholars Publishing

The Elixir of Platelet Rich Plasma Therapy in Intervention Dermatology and Regenerative Trichology

Edited by Suruchi Garg

This book first published 2023

Cambridge Scholars Publishing

Lady Stephenson Library, Newcastle upon Tyne, NE6 2PA, UK

British Library Cataloguing in Publication Data
A catalogue record for this book is available from the British Library

ISBN (10): 1-5275-1072-7
ISBN (13): 978-1-5275-1072-2

TABLE OF CONTENTS

CONTRIBUTORS

Dr. Suruchi Garg MD
Founder Director and Chief Consultant Dermatologist, Aura Skin Institute, Chandigarh

Dr. Anuva Bansal MD
Consultant Dermatologist, BLK-MAX Super Specialty Hospital & AB Centre for Skin and Hair, New Delhi

Ms. Kashvi Garg
Senior secondary school medical student, Carmel Convent School, Chandigarh

Dr. Shweta Manchanda MD
Consultant Dermatologist Skinkarma, Delhi

Dr Lakkireddygari Sujana MD
Assistant professor, Prathima institute of medical sciences, Karimnagar, Telangana

Dr. Carol Lobo MD
Senior Resident - St John's Medical College Hospital, Banglore

Dr Jill Chitalia MD (dermatology), FMUHS(Tricho), FIADVl (lasers and aesthetics). Co-founder and Business head, Skinnsi, Mumbai

Dr. Ankita Tuknayat MD
Senior Resident, Department of Dermatology, Government Medical College and Hospital, Chandigarh

Dr. Rubina Alves MD, PhD
Specialist in Dermatology and Venereology, Instituto Dermatológico da Madeira, Portugal

Dr Shreya Agarwal MD
Co-founder & Consultant Dermatologist, Gupta Lifecare Hospital, Hanumangarh, Rajasthan

Dr Trusha Mistry MD
Consultant Dermatologist, RIMS Superspeciality Hospital, Ghdasar, Ahmedabad

Dr. Aayushi Shah MD
Consultant Dermatologist, Navkar Surgical Hospital, Ahmedabad.

Dr. Shefali Porwal MD
Consultant, Department of Dermatology, Medanta Hospital and Research Institute, Lucknow, U.P.

Dr Devi Menon
Consultant Dermatologist, Dr. Yogiraj Centre for Dermatology and Cosmetology, Trivendrum, Kerala

Dr. Ami Badheka MD
Consultant Clinical and Cosmetic Dermatologist, Parli Cosmetic and Laser Centre, Ahmedabad

FOREWORD

Dr Suruchi Garg has focused on treating dermatologic and genetic conditions that cause hair loss for many years. Her interest in this field was apparent when she visited my clinic years ago and since then has developed a special interest in regenerative medicine and specifically in the potential that platelet-rich plasma (PRP) has in treating the disorders causing hair loss.

In this book the readers will find the theoretical and practical, the science and the art, all carefully blended for the benefit of the readers. It is clear that Dr Garg is an advocate for using the unique properties of the human biological system to treat various conditions, and this book explains how PRP can be of benefit. When relevant, she provides the studies to support the use of PRP in certain situations and then offers the practical knowledge required to deliver the treatment.

If you treat hair loss and you want to provide PRP to your patients, you will find Dr Garg's book to be thorough and practical and it will allow you to deliver this therapy in a safe and effective manner.

James A. Harris, MD, FISHRS
Medical Director – RESTORE
Hair Restoration and Transplant
Chicago, United States
Hair Science Centre, Greenwood Village, Colorado,
United States

******

The passion for regenerative medicine and for the treatment of some pathologies addressed by it, such as alopecia, has led over the years many scientists to better investigate, through rigorous scientific studies, the possible new autologous therapies in the treatment of hair loss.

All the latest knowledge in the treatment of alopecia using platelet-rich plasma reported by all the experts who have decided to contribute to the realization of this work deserves to be read.

Pietro Gentile, MD, PhD
Associate Professor of Plastic and Reconstructive Surgery
University of Rome "Tor Vergata"
Regenerative Surgery PhD
Top Italian Scientist (H-Index >31)

******

Platelet-rich plasma (PRP) contains several growth factors and cellular adhesion molecules which promote wound healing, angiogenesis and accelerate the rejuvenation of skin and hair follicles. With its proven regenerative and regrowth potential in a plethora of conditions.

Use of PRP alone or in combination with hair transplant in androgenetic alopecia is well-researched indication. It has shown excellent results when utilized in combination with microneedling or ablative lasers in acne scars, post-burn or post-traumatic scars, melasma, striae distensae, chronic ulcers and lichen sclerosis. PRP injections or PRP combined with microneedling are increasingly being utilized for skin rejuvenation and recently have been utilized to provide non-invasive face lifts. Combining non-cultured epidermal cell suspension suspended in PRP results in superior re-pigmentation outcomes in case of vitiligo. PRP has now become an indispensable tool in the dermatology practitioner's armamentarium and a comprehensive text covering all the relevant aspects regarding this therapy was the need of the hour. Though there are a lot of articles available on PRP, each article mentions some different protocol and method creating a great deal of confusion among the readers.

This all-inclusive textbook discusses the various indications, techniques, modifications of PRP as well as its application in various indications in great detail with special mention of the practical aspects.

The book shall be a ready reckoner for the practicing dermatologists, dermatosurgeons, general surgeons, plastic surgeons and other clinicians who are fascinated by this novel technique. It will be a go to book for all your queries regarding PRP.

I wish all the very best to the editor who has great experience in effectively utilizing this "wonder tool" in interventional dermatology as well as trichology. She has previously published several novel research articles and this textbook is an amalgamation of her expertise, knowledge and practical understanding of PRP along with the contributions of leading dermatologists who put in hard work to compile the current knowledge, besides contributing their thoughts and ideas regarding these diverse aspects.

I am sure that this book will be widely received and acclaimed.

Dr Rachita Dhurat
Organizing Chairperson, Trichology Update
Professor & Head of Department of Dermatology
LTM Medical College & Hospital Sion,
Mumbai 400022

******

Dermatology is a vast subject which is continuously in a state of evolution. Besides medical dermatology, dermatosurgery and cosmetic dermatology are rapidly growing. Platelet-rich plasma (PRP) therapy is a modality which is being used for several dermatological diseases and the evidence is gradually accumulating. Dr Suruchi Garg is a well-known dermatology practitioner with several publications to her credit and has now produced this multi-authored book on PRP. This book will be a handy reckoner to both early and senior practitioners who use physical modalities in their practice. I would like to congratulate her and all the authors for writing on different aspects of treatment of skin disorders with PRP. I wish the editor luck for her well-intentioned book and happy reading to the interested readers.

Dr Rashmi Sarkar MD FAMS,
Director Professor of Dermatology,
Lady Hardinge Medical College and Associated Hospitals,
New Delhi, India
President, Indian Association of Dermatologists, Venereologists and
Leprologists (IADVL) 2022

******

Platelet-rich plasma (PRP) is autologous concentration of platelets contained in small volume of plasma which accelerates the rejuvenation of skin and hair follicles (HFs) due to presence of various growth factors and cellular adhesion molecules. PRP therapy is a relatively new approach to tissue regeneration, which is becoming a valuable adjunct to promote healing and enhance treatment outcomes of various procedures in medical and surgical fields.

Over the last decade, PRP has attained a well-deserved place in the therapeutic armamentarium of dermatologists in variety of indications including hair loss, post-acne scarring, disorders of pigmentation, non-healing ulcers, facial rejuvenation, and regenerative medicine. Apart from dermatology and aesthetic practice, it is increasingly being used in maxillofacial surgery, periodontal and oral medicine, otolaryngology, orthopaedic and trauma, cardiovascular, gastrointestinal, burns, and plastic surgery. While there is growing popularity of PRP among dermatologists and other specialities, a scarcity is felt for textbooks and evidence-based standardized protocols on the science of PRP. Dr Suruchi Garg is one of the leading experts from India who has extensively used and pioneered art of PRP in dermatology and aesthetic medicine practice. Dr Suruchi Garg and her co-authors have filled this void through their enriching contribution.

This textbook provides an excellent learning and reference material across the whole spectrum of the use of PRP. It is going to be an asset for young dermatologists and postgraduate students who wish to learn and incorporate PRP in their practice. I would highly recommend it for anyone who is interested in obtaining basic knowledge of PRP, research, or updating and perfecting existing knowledge and skills.

I congratulate Dr Suruchi Garg for her vision, conviction, dedication, and all the hard work in bringing out this excellent textbook.

Sunil Dogra
MD, DNB, FAMS, FAAD, Dip. Dermatology (Glasgow), FRCP (London)
FRCP (Edinburgh)
Professor, Department of Dermatology, Venereology & Leprology
Postgraduate Institute of Medical Education & Research (PGIMER)
Chandigarh, 160012, India
Editor Emeritus: Indian Dermatology Online Journal

PREFACE

The insatiable curiosity of the human mind constantly motivates it to improve the existing treatment modalities and has led to path-breaking discoveries and inventions. While many researchers toil hard in labs – discovering and establishing the role of new drugs and formulations; others are fascinated by the body's own healing capacity and ability to regenerate it. This is what essentially lays down the foundation of regenerative medicine.

Regenerative medicine is an upcoming branch where the body's own cells, tissues, or fluids can be regenerated, engineered or replaced to restore and establish normal functions. Platelet-rich plasma is one such promising therapy that is increasingly being utilized as an adjunct to standard medical and surgical therapies and is expected to be the future of various regenerative and restorative therapies.

This book aims at bringing forth the most innovative and minimally invasive techniques, to improve the outcome of existing diseases and to improve the tell-tale signs of burned-out diseases through PRP cocktails. PRP therapy has gained immense popularity in the past decade in the field of intervention dermatology and regenerative trichology, but there are a lot of trials and tribulations making the subject all the more intriguing and difficult to understand. Detailed and organized research work is the need of the hour to bring more clarity to the subject for researchers, clinicians and practitioners working in this field.

This book is written and compiled based on the existing literature on PRP therapy along with excerpts from my own personal experiences and publications in different journals over 10 years.

It will discuss at length the methods of preparation of PRP, single spin versus double spin, role in different types of alopecia, hair transplant and scarring alopecia, scar management, pigmentary disorders, facial rejuvenation and non-healing ulcers. There will also be a mention of the use of novel surgeries like our innovative vitiligo surgery called LA-PEEST (laser ablation of recipient area with PRP-enriched epidermal-dermal suspension transplant) and RA-PEEST (radiofrequency ablation with PRP-enriched epidermal-dermal suspension transplant) aimed at making new skin, which would otherwise heal with secondary intention and possibly scarring.

Towards the end, very passionately and ambitiously we discuss the use of various live cells including hair follicle-derived stem cells which are the future of regenerative therapy, as treatment options for various ailments in intervention dermatology and regenerative trichology.

In various academic forums, one sees a vast majority of clinicians not entirely convinced about the efficacy of platelet-rich plasma in spite of the plethora of literature supporting its mechanism of action and results. Along similar lines, there is another set of clinicians, who believe that nutrition and correction of underlying deficiencies do not offer many roles in modifying a disease process.

In my humble opinion, both regenerative medicine and nutrigenomics lay down the foundation of future medicine, and together they lay down the foundation to a very crucial and synergistic role to be played to facilitate the healing process. It is analogous to supporting the "organic and green approach" instead of "industrialized management of disease pathogenesis" inside the human body. Endorsing the same understanding in my practice, we have very passionately pursued and observed the role of both nutrition and regenerative medicine working hand in glove. At the end of the day, researchers and clinicians need to understand the biology, chemistry and dynamics of the body's signals being generated at the cellular level. The response is based on the type of substrate available; in turn, the response of the tissues, organs and systems is based on circadian rhythm and endocrine, paracrine, autocrine and enzymatic signals dictating the course of action towards healing or inflammation. It is astonishing to observe that the injuries on these sites can be healed and modified with additional growth factors released from platelet-rich plasma and other regenerative tissues, kick-starting an array of chemical reactions and cascade of events to aid the healing process and improve the overall environment. The current work in regenerative medicine is just the beginning of a highly fruitful and fulfilling journey and hopefully, more researchers will be benefited and inspired to explore the vast ocean of knowledge in this direction.

The purpose of bringing out this book is to bridge the gap between existing medical treatments and the body's regenerative capacity through regenerative medicine and to create an understanding of utilizing the body's own immense healing potential. This book provides a concise and result-oriented approach to the field of regenerative medicine and interestingly, some of the major work described is based on cocktail treatments, which hasten the results in fewer sessions without compromising the patient's safety. The work should interest all those physicians and surgeons who believe in providing minimally invasive procedures, which eventually create a significant difference in their patients' quality of life. The approach has the potential to provide hope to patients suffering from recalcitrant diseases, otherwise not amenable to conventional dermatology treatments.

Dr Suruchi Garg

INTRODUCTION

Dr Suruchi Garg is the Director and Chief Consultant at Aura Skin Institute, Chandigarh, India. She was awarded her MBBS from IGMC Shimla, a premier institute located in the lap of Himalayas and post-graduation in dermatology from one of India's most coveted and prestigious tertiary care institute, the Post Graduate Institute of Medical Education and Research (PGIMER), Chandigarh.

Dr Garg has undertaken advanced training in lasers from Cesaria, Israel and hair transplant training from Denver, US. She won a Young Dermatologist Forum Award for her work on cutaneous vasculitis in the most prestigious national conference, Dermacon 2008. She was also honoured with the Distinguished Scholar Award 2020 by the European Journal of Scientific Research for her outstanding contribution for the use of platelet-rich plasma therapy and hair transplant in the field of scarring alopecia. Besides this, she has numerous state and national level awards, and accolades to her credit for bringing in the latest cutting-edge technologies and innovations in the field of intervention dermatology and regenerative trichology.

Dr Garg is the programme director for IADVL (Indian Association of Dermatologists, Venereologists and Leprologists) with a fellowship in lasers and aesthetics, and specializes in training post-dermatology fellows in lasers, vitiligo surgeries, hair transplant, platelet-rich plasma, and various aesthetic procedures. She has innovated a surgical technique in vitiligo patients (LA-PEEST) which delivers faster re-pigmentation and aesthetically more acceptable results, as published in the international journal Dermatologic Surgery. She has performed numerous such surgeries to reduce the psychological impact and the disease burden in scores of vitiligo patients.

She has filed patents in non–surgical facelift through fat repositioning and another on an AI (artificial intelligence) based approach aimed in the same direction, which she genuinely considers "a step towards true anti-ageing". According to her, the approach can minimize the use of external fillers as it utilizes the patient's own facial droopy fat planes. Dr Garg has also proposed and published a global drooping and wrinkle (DW) classification for facial age estimation. She is undergoing pioneering work in regenerative medicine with publications in various national and international journals and books of high repute, and conducting training courses and workshops at national and international levels.

Dr Garg has been designated the key opinion leader (KOL) by many companies of international repute such as Alma and BTL aesthetics. She is actively contributing to innovation and technology with maximum safety and efficacy for the treatment of Asian skin types. She is also a passionate nutritionist and has various papers on nutrition, skin and hair disorders, and has also conceptualized a protein-based health supplement based on the "principle of circadian rhythm and science of proteins". Currently, she is the section editor for Indian Dermatology Online Journal and a member of editorial team in the journal *Cosmoderma,* and a reviewer for various other prestigious international journals.

CHAPTER 1

THE HISTORY OF BLOOD, BLOOD PRODUCTS AND THEIR USES SINCE ANCIENT TIMES

SURUCHI GARG, KASHVI GARG, ANUVA BANSAL

"*We are linked by blood, and blood is memory without language*"
—Joyce Carol Oates

Blood is mysteriously being chased in incantations, potions, religious practices, medieval medical treatises and works of fiction. The Ebers papyrus, the ancient Egyptian literature is written in hieratic Egyptian language. It is based on elaborate medical knowledge transferred through pre-existing literature and dates back to 1500 BC.[1] It mentions the heart as the centre of blood supply and various vessels linking the heart to every organ of the body. The prevalent "channel theory" proclaimed unimpeded blood flow to different organs of the body as the essential prerequisite for good health. In the Indian subcontinent, the era of establishing the role of blood and its components goes back to more than 600 BC with the meticulous scrutiny of the available literature. The first manuscripts are written in Sanskrit, the most ancient language of the world often touted as the mother of all languages. These manuscripts are *Sushruta Samhita, Charaka Samhita, Bala Samhita* and so many more written by the eminent Ayurvedic physicians and surgeons in those times. The *Charaka Samhita* deals with medicine, written by famous Ayurvedic physician Charaka and describes in depth the circulatory system (*Rasavaha srotas*) in the body and suggests that the system works like a rotating wheel.[2] Sushruta (around 600 BC) in his primeval compendium *Sushruta Samhita* mentioned that the pattern of blood flow was identical to the velocity of sound, fire and water, which are maximum at the source and gradually diminish away from the source or heart.[3] Sushruta, a renowned plastic surgeon in those times is regarded as the *father of plastic surgery* in the ancient Indian medical system. He is known to have had excellent knowledge about the circulatory system and it is mentioned in the compendium that his knowledge was principally derived by conducting the post mortems of dead bodies floating in the water, passed on to him by his teachers.[3] As per Ayurvedic literature, there are four components of blood: 1) "Rasa" or plasma, the nutrient fluid that nourishes the rest of the tissues; 2) "Rakta", the red fraction (red blood cells) that is essential for life; 3) "Ojas", a white fraction (white blood cells and platelets), the functions of which are closely associated with immunity; and 4) "Prana", (oxygen) a fraction that is derived through the act of respiration. Therefore, the tissue that is today known as "blood" should include all these components.[4]

Knowledge in the ancient world

In the ancient world, the function of the heart and vessels were a great mystery. Many hundred years BC the Greeks Herophilus of Chalcedon (c. 335 to c. 260 BC) and Alcamaeon of Croton (c. 535 to unknown BC) believed that arteries and veins are dissimilar in animals when compared to those of humans; they believed that arteries are thicker than veins and distribute the blood.[5] There is a possibility of various interactions having taken place between the scholars of ancient Greece and India, especially when Alexander the Great (326 BC) invaded India, specifically the places around Taxila, one of the ancient seats of learning.[6] Eventual outcomes could have been the mixing of information and both sides influencing and contributing to existing knowledge.

The Greeks described the presence of erythrocytes (red blood cells) in blood, giving it the characteristic colour. According to the most widespread ancient Greek scientific views, the blood was believed to be a necessary nutrient of the living body, as are juices for plants.

Hippocrates (450–380 BC) knew that blood moves and performs a periodic or circular movement – *"periodon, cyclon"*.[7] He also believed that blood is produced in the liver and spleen and travels to the heart, and is warmed or cooled in the lungs. There was also existing knowledge that the human body has four types of fluid (blood, phlegm, and black and yellow bile).[8]

Aristotle (384–322 BC) considered blood to be the essence of nutrition and the preserver of body heat, and termed it the ultimate food. Blood is the food in its most perfect form, which creates and preserves the noblest parts of the body – the flesh and other sensory organs.[9]

According to Claudius Galenus of Pergamon (200–130 BC) *hema* is a warm and fluid material that is present in the arteries, from which the animal is fed.[10] Galenus's words *haema einai ten psychen* meaning blood is the soul were a few of the misleading beliefs in those times. Galenus also believed that life was sustained by food, which turned into blood in the liver, which nourished the lungs, heart, brain and other organs along with the removal of waste products. Thus, blood circulation and metabolism became the significant elements of his philosophical theory, and he was a pioneer in suggesting a relationship between food, blood and air.[10,11]

Later discoveries

Subsequent centuries saw landmark discoveries related to circulatory systems such as the discovery of the existence of heart valves (Iranian Rhazes, AD 865–925) and pulmonary circulation (Syrian Ibn Al-Nafis, AD 1210–1288).[12,13]

The British scientist William Harvey (1627) showed that blood circulated within a closed circuit. He is credited with suggesting a robust mathematical model of the motion of heart and blood in animals, and described the mechanisms of both systemic and pulmonary circulation in humans.[14]

The German (Franz) Ernst Neuman (1866) demonstrated clearly that nucleated erythropoiesis and leukopoiesis formulate in the bone marrow. He also became the first person to postulate the bone marrow as a blood-forming organ with a common stem cell for all haematopoietic cells.[15] The British scientist William Osler (1870) made the first description of *platelets*, explained the formation of blood clots and hinted at possible synthesis in the bone marrow. The British surgeon William Hewson (1869), who noted that the red cells were flat rather than globular and described the leukocytes for the first time, has been referred to as the *father of haematology*.[16]

The first documented blood transfusion to a human from a sheep was administered by the Frenchman Jean-Baptiste Denis (1667) and the first human-to-human transfusion was performed by British obstetrician James Blundell (1818).[4,15,16] The Austrian Karl Landsteiner (1901) documented the three human blood groups (A, B and O) for the first time, and subsequently the American Reuben Ottenberg (1907) is credited for performing the first blood transfusion using blood typing and cross-matching.[12,17,18]

The first report of the application of native blood in wound treatment was recorded in 1876 in Germany, and it was noticed that wounds healed quickly. In 1898 in the USA, autologous blood mixed with normal saline was used to treat pneumonia and tuberculosis. Reports of accelerated broken bone recovery and consolidation by 30% with the patient's own blood injections in the thigh came from German surgeon August Bier. The method of autohaemotherapy in "nidus of inflammation and infections" such as furuncles and carbuncles in *Purulent surgery assays* was reported in 1934 by Russian surgeon Valentine Voino-Yasenetsky.

Platelet-rich plasma

The terminology, platelet-rich plasma, was used by C. S. Kinsley in 1954[19] to refer to platelet concentrate for transfusion. Subsequently, the various growth factors were detected in platelet-rich plasma aiding the healing process. In the late 1990s Marx et al. pioneered the usage of plasma in the form of gel clots mainly for the repair of bone defects in dental surgeries.[19-21] These case reports were the dawn of the new era of regenerative medicine in the late twentieth and early twenty-first century. Subsequently, the journey of blood embarked upon the healing of wounds, injuries and complicated non-responsive-delayed healing disorders in different streams of orthopaedics, sports medicine, dentistry, dermatology and plastic surgery.

In our humble journey of utilizing platelet-rich plasma in intervention dermatology and regenerative trichology, we observed its great healing potential and termed it an "elixir", provided it is used in the right direction with an adequate supply of nutrition creating the right environment for healing.[22,23] Thus, our approach almost comes full circle with the history of blood, with the Galenus philosophy suggesting a relationship between blood, food and air. It suggests strong interdependence of blood, nutrition and inner well-being to attain the desired results.

> But all these requisites belong of old to Medicine, and an origin and way have been found out, by which many and elegant discoveries have been made, during a length of time, and others will yet be found out, if a person possessed of the proper ability, and knowing those discoveries which have been made, should proceed from them to prosecute his investigations.
> (Hippocrates, *On Ancient Medicine*)

References

1. Stern LC (1875), Ebers G, editors. Papyros Ebers: Das hermetische Buch über die Arzeneimittel der alten Ägypter in hieratischer Schrift, herausgegeben mit Inhaltsangabe und Einleitung versehen von Georg Ebers, mit Hieroglyphisch-Lateinischem Glossar von Ludwig Stern,

mit Unterstützung des Königlich Sächsischen Cultusministerium (in German). Vol. 2. Leipzig: W. Englemann. LCCN 25012078. Retrieved 18 September 2010.

2. Pandey G, editor. The Caraka Samhita of Agnivesha (5th ed.). Varanasi, India: Chaukhambha Sanskrit Sansthan: 2006. Vols. 1 and 2: The Kashi Sanskrit series no. 194.
3. Acharya JT, editor. Sushruta Samhita of Sushruta. Varanasi, India: Chaukhambha Surbharati Prakashan: 1994. The Chaukhmbha Ayurvijnan Granthamala No 42.
4. Patwardhan K. The history of the discovery of blood circulation: unrecognized contributions of Ayurveda masters. *Adv Physiol Educ*. 2012;**36**:77-82.
5. Ducasse E, Speziale F, Baste JC, Midy D. Vascular knowledge in medieval times was the turning point for the humanistic trend. *Eur J Vasc Endovasc Surg*. 2006;**31**:600-608.
6. Aziz W. Taxila: a meeting ground of nations. In: Sharma SK, Sharma U, editors. Encyclopaedia of higher education: the Indian perspective. New Delhi, India: Mittal; 2005, vol. 1.
7. Jouanna J, Hippocrate. Paris, France: Fayard;1992.
8. Shoja MM, Tubbs RS, Loukas M, Ardalan MR. The Aristotelian account of "heart and veins", *Int J Cardiol*. 2008;**125**:304-310.
9. Barnes J, *The Complete Work of Aristotle: The Revised Oxford Translation*, Princeton University Press, Princeton (NJ): 1984.
10. Hankinson R, The man and his work. In: Hankinson R, editor. The Cambridge Companion to Galen (Cambridge Companions to Philosophy) Cambridge: Cambridge University Press; 2008. p. 1-33. doi:10.1017/CCOL9780521819541.001
11. Meletis J, Konstantopoulos K. The beliefs, myths, and reality surrounding the word hema (blood) from Homer to the present. *Anemia*. 2010;2010:857657. https://doi.org/10.1155/2010/857657
12. Azizi M-H, Nayernouri T, Azizi F. A brief history of the discovery of the circulation of blood in the human body. *Arch Iran Med*. 2008;**11**:345-350.
13. Loukas M, Lam R, Tubbs RS, Shoja MAM, Apaydin N. Ibn al-Nafis (1210–1288): the first description of the pulmonary circulation. *Am Surg*. 2008;**74**:440-442.
14. Harvey W. On the motion of the heart and blood in animals, translated by Willis R. New York: NY: Prometheus, 1993.
15. Zech NH, Shkumatov A, Koestenbauer S. The magic behind stem cells. *J Assist Reprod Genet*. 2007;**24**:208-214.

16. Kleinzeller A. William Hewson's studies of red blood corpuscles and the evolving concept of a cell membrane. *Am J Physiol*. 1996;**271**:C1–C8, 1996.
17. Khan IA, Daya SK, Gowda, RM. Evolution of the theory of circulation. *Int J Cardiol.* 2005;**98**:519-521.
18. Tan SY, Graham C. Karl Landsteiner (1868–1943): originator of ABO blood classification. Singapore Med J. 2013;54:243-244. doi: 10.11622/smedj.2013099.
19. Masic I, Dilic M, Solakovic E, Rustempasic N, Ridjanovic Z. Why historians of medicine called Ibn al-Nafis second Avicenna? *Med Arh.* 2008;**62**:244-249.
20. Marx RE, Carlson ER, Eichstaedt RM, Schimmele SR, Strauss JE, Georgeff KR. Platelet-rich plasma: growth factor enhancement for bone grafts. *Oral Surg Oral Med Oral Pathol Oral Radiol Endod.* 1998 Jun;**85**:638-46. doi: 10.1016/s1079-2104(98)90029-4.
21. Anitua E. Plasma rich in growth factors: preliminary results of use in the preparation of future sites for implants. *Int J Oral Maxillofac Implants.* 1999 Jul-Aug;**14**:529-35. PMID: 10453668.
22. Marx RE. Platelet-rich plasma (PRP): what is PRP and what is not PRP? *Implant Dent*. 2001;**10**:225-228.
23. Garg S, Manchanda S. Platelet-rich plasma – an "elixir" for treatment of alopecia: personal experience on 117 patients with review of literature. *Stem Cell Investig*. 2017;**4**:64. doi:10.21037/sci.2017.06.07
24. Garg S, Bansal A. Platelet-rich plasma in interventional dermatology and trichology: How far have we come? *Cosmoderma*. 2021;**1**:2.

CHAPTER 2

DIFFERENT TYPES OF PRP AND METHODS OF PREPARATION

SHWETA MANCHANDA, ANUVA BANSAL, SURUCHI GARG

Introduction

Platelet-rich plasma (PRP) is defined as an autologous blood-derived product enriched in platelets, growth factors and chemo/cytokines which are delivered in a concentrated volume of plasma. Since the 1970s, PRP has received significant attention in the field of tissue repair and regeneration. Initial studies focused mainly on applications within the musculoskeletal and maxillofacial fields; however, now it is being used for various dermatological indications including wound healing, fat grafting, alopecia and scar management, as well as soft tissue volume augmentation.[1]

Synonyms: autologous platelet gel, plasma-rich growth factors, platelet-concentrated plasma, platelet-rich concentrate, platelet release.[2]

It is the volume of the plasma fraction of autologous blood having an above-baseline platelet concentration (more than 1,000,000 platelets/µl) thereby leading to 300%–700% enrichment.[2,3]

Concentration of platelets

Platelet concentration is the most frequently described parameter and it primarily influences the efficacy of PRP. A concentration of two to six times higher than the basal platelet count is required for optimal outcomes.[4]

Whole blood consists of 93% red blood cells, 6% platelets and 1% white blood cells. In PRP, the proportion of these cells in blood is reversed. The red cell layer is reduced to 5%, and platelets and leukocytes are increased to about 94% to stimulate tissue regeneration.[5]

Normal platelet count in blood ranges between 150,000 and 400,000 platelets/µl, and average platelet count is 200,000 ±75,000/µl. A platelet concentration of more than 1 million/µl (approximately four to seven times the mean levels) in a 5 ml volume of plasma is the working definition and therapeutically effective concentration of PRP. Lesser concentrations cannot be relied upon to enhance wound healing, and greater concentrations have not been shown to increase wound healing.[6-8]

Rughetti et al. in their study found the relationship between the platelet concentration in platelet gel and changes in the functional activity of human endothelial cells. The endothelial cell proliferation, migration and invasion occurred in a bell-shaped manner indicating a dose-dependent nature. They found that the stimulation for endothelial cell proliferation peaks at 1.25 × 106 and angiogenesis at 1.5 × 106 platelets/ml, respectively.[9]

Giusti et al. stated that lower or higher concentrations than 1.5 million platelets/µl inhibit the angiogenic potential in human endothelial cells. In vitro dermal papilla cell studies have also supported PRP concentrations of five to ten times the mean levels.[6]

Mazzucco et al. suggested that a platelet count of more than 2 × 105/µl may be sufficient for therapeutic effect.[10] Gentile et al. concluded that a mean of 1.48 million platelets per microlitre stimulated follicular and perifollicular angiogenesis, which led to active hair growth.[11]

Qualitative changes in the platelets also affect the regenerative potential of PRP. According to Marx, a damaged or non-viable platelet will not lead to the release of bioactive growth factors, thus the resulting PRP may not be effective.[3] The platelets actively secrete growth factors within 10 minutes of activation and more than 95% of the pre-synthesized growth factors are secreted within 1 hour.[2]

Therefore, PRP should be used within 10 minutes of activation. The viability of the concentrated platelets remains for up to 8 hours and they remain sterile if placed on a sterile surgical table.[2]

The platelets remain viable for 7–10 days and the release of growth factors in the tissue continues during this period.[2] Thus, a good PRP device should process a concentration of at least 1,000,000 platelets/µl in a 5-ml volume with viable undamaged platelets in a sterile environment, and the resultant PRP should be pyrogen-free.[7]

Principles of PRP preparation

PRP is prepared by the process of differential centrifugation. In differential centrifugation, acceleration force is adjusted so there is the sedimentation of certain cellular constituents based on different specific gravity.[12] A 30-cc venous blood draw yields 3–5 cc of PRP depending on the baseline platelet count of an individual, the device used and the technique employed.[12]

PRP is prepared either manually, or using automated devices or kits.[1] In the manual method, blood is withdrawn from the patient, an anticoagulant is added and the mixture is centrifuged without using any automated device or kit. The manual method can be double spin or single spin.[1]

Manual double-spin method

The American Association of Blood Banks technical manual states that "platelet-rich plasma is separated from whole blood by 'light-spin' centrifugation and the platelets are subsequently concentrated by 'heavy-spin' centrifugation with the removal of the supernatant plasma".[13]

The centrifugation process separates blood components depending on their different specific gravities, i.e. red blood cells (RBCs) being the heaviest followed by white blood cells (WBCs), whereas platelets are the lightest. The first centrifugation is slow to avoid spinning down the platelets and isolating plasma. Platelets are mainly concentrated right on top of the buffy coat layer. Subsequent centrifugation is faster so that platelets are spun down and are separated as a pellet at the bottom of the tube from platelet-poor plasma (PPP) above. The final platelet concentration depends on the volume reduction of the PPP. Approximately three-quarters of the supernatant is discarded and the platelet-rich pellet is re-suspended in the remaining quarter of plasma. The resulting suspension is PRP.[6] (Figure 1)

Calcium chloride ($CaCl2$) or thrombin can be used as an activator to trigger coagulation and therefore lead to degranulation of growth factors to yield activated PRP.[6]

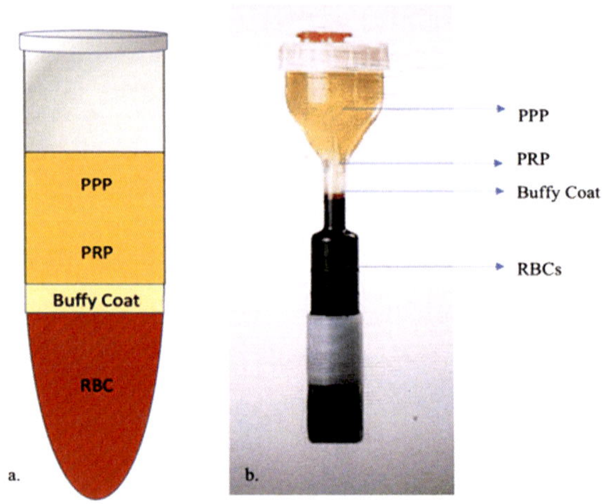

Figure 1: Components of PRP: a. Normal acid citrate dextrose (ACD) vial; b. Hourglass tube: in the single-spin method, the lower portion of the plasma layer is collected as PRP. To increase the platelet concentration of PRP, the plasma and superficial buffy coat can be collected, and a second centrifugation can be performed. PPP, platelet-poor plasma; P-PRP, pure platelet-rich plasma; RBC, red blood cells.

Double or single spin?

The value of the second centrifugation relates to the concept that after a single spin, the RBCs interfere with the fine separation of the platelets regardless of the rate or the time of centrifugation, thus producing a preparation with a smaller percentage of PRP.[1] The double-spin method is preferred over the single-spin method, as it not possible to separate and concentrate platelets to a therapeutic level with only the single-spin method.[14-16] The first centrifugation is aimed to separate RBC from other segments of the whole blood. As RBC is red, visible and heavy in specific gravity, the best condition is the lowest and shortest speed and time at which RBC and plasma can be easily separated visibly. Too much speed and time will let platelets also precipitate and should be avoided, hence 230–270g for 10 minutes is reported to be the most efficient for the first centrifugation.[15]

As the second centrifugation is aimed to separate platelets from plasma, the speed and time should be as high and as long as permissible to avoid alteration in platelet morphology. Doing this at a higher speed and for longer period of time will lead to the precipitation of more platelets.[15]

Marx et al. noted that regardless of the rate or the time of centrifugation, a single spin cannot adequately concentrate platelets, because the red blood cells will interfere with the fine separation of the platelets.[7]

Methods of producing PRP

There are two principal methods of PRP production – the PRP method and the buffy coat method.[12,17]

The PRP method uses fresh blood from venepuncture, which is centrifuged for a "soft" spin to separate the red blood cells (RBCs). The supernatant plasma is then centrifuged in a "hard" spin at higher speeds to obtain the platelet concentrate.[17]

The first spin is done at constant acceleration to separate RBCs from the remaining whole blood (WB) volume. After the first spin step, the WB separates into three layers: an upper layer that contains mostly platelets and WBC, an intermediate thin layer that is the buffy coat and is rich in WBCs, and a bottom layer that consists mainly of RBCs. The upper layer and superficial buffy coat are transferred to an empty sterile tube. The "g" for the second spin must be just adequate, and thus aid the formation of soft pellets (erythrocyte-platelet) at the bottom of the tube.[12,17]

The buffy coat technique utilizes whole blood, pre-stored at room temperature (i.e. 20–24°C). It undergoes a "hard" spin to separate it into three layers: RBCs, platelets and white blood cells (WBCs), and platelet-poor plasma. The supernatant plasma is removed and the buffy coat is separated. This layer undergoes a second low-speed spin to separate the WBCs, or a leukocyte filter can be used.[17] A buffy coat contains a high concentration of leukocytes. From the small volume of WB (10 ml), a very thin layer of a buffy coat can be produced. The difficulty lies in separating this thin buffy coat layer that contains mainly WBCs and platelets from the underlying RBC layer.[12,17]

a) PRP method[14]

- Whole blood is collected by venipuncture in ACD tubes.
- Blood is not chilled at any time before or during platelet separation.
- Blood is centrifuged using a soft spin.
- Supernatant plasma containing platelets is transferred into another sterile tube (without anticoagulant).

- The second tube is centrifuged at a higher speed (hard spin) to obtain a platelet concentrate.
- The lower one-third is PRP, and the upper two-thirds is called platelet-poor plasma. Platelet pellets are formed at the bottom of the tube.
- PPP is removed, and the platelet pellet is suspended in a minimum quantity of plasma (2–4 ml) by gently shaking the tube.

b) Buffy coat method[14]

- Whole blood is stored at 20–24°C before centrifugation.
- After storage, blood is centrifuged at a high speed.
- Three layers are formed because of the density: the bottom layer consists of RBCs, the middle layer consists of platelets and WBCs and the top layer is the PPP.
- Supernatant plasma is removed from the top of the container.
- The buffy coat layer is transferred to another sterile tube.
- It is centrifuged at low speed to separate WBCs, or a leukocyte filtration filter is used.[17]

Automated devices

Numerous automated devices and kits of varying standards have been manufactured in the last few years to facilitate the delivery of ready-to-apply PRP without the need for manual separation. The limitation associated with the available commercial devices is that their products are likely to have potentially dissimilar biology, which leads to challenges in comparing clinical efficacy.[1]

Though automated devices are more convenient to use and quicker compared to manual methods, they are also more expensive.[10]

Commercial interests also obscure the true clinical benefits of various platelet concentrates. The easy reproducibility of the product is not consistent with the devices and kits. A prudent clinician needs to ensure the viability, concentration and activation of platelets obtained by these devices.[6]

PRP devices can be divided into lower (2.5–3 times baseline concentration) and higher (5–9 times baseline concentration) systems. The high-yielding devices are the Zimmer Biomet GPS II® and III® (platelet count 3–8 times); Harvest SmartPreP® 2 APC+™ (4–6 times); Arteriocyte-Medtronic Magellan (3–7 times). The lower concentration systems comprise Arthrex ACP® (2–3 times), Cascade® PRP therapy (1–1.5

times), PRGF® by the BTI Biotechnology Institute in Vitoria-Gasteiz, Spain (2–3 times) and RegenPRP® (Regen Laboratory, Le Mont-sur-Lausanne, Switzerland).[12] Some of the kits have been approved by the US Food and Drug Association (FDA), such as SmartPreP® (Harvest Technologies Inc, Plymouth, MA, USA), PCCS® (3i Implant Innovations Inc, Palm Beach Gardens, FL, USA) and Zimmer4 BioMet GPS II®.[1]

Our method

We use the Renew Cell Kit and the Remi cold centrifuge for the preparation of PRP. Two vials, each containing 10 ml of whole blood mixed with 1.5 ml of ACD-A solution are used and centrifuged for four minutes at 3,400 rpm (revolutions per minute) with 1,350 RCF (relative centrifugal force). Out of these two vials, a total of 4–5 ml of the buffy coat along with PRP is harvested and injected as per requirement. It gives nearly three times the concentration of the baseline platelet count, though for higher concentrations the volume of plasma can be reduced, which yields a higher concentration of platelets.

Comparison of preparation protocols

Numerous protocols have attempted to optimize the centrifugation procedure using different performance standards and centrifugation parameters.[18]

However, the various protocols have been optimized with respect to different variables such as volume and sampling of processed WB, number of spins, centrifugation time and the range of centrifugal acceleration.[12]

Arora et al. studied different double centrifugation protocols. They noticed that when the centrifugation time increased, the platelet concentration became higher. The highest platelet concentration was after the first centrifugation at 440 g for 20 minutes. They investigated the release rate of different growth factors and concluded that the best protocol was 208 g for 20 minutes, because increasing the centrifugation force led to platelet aggregation and a faulty release of growth factors.[19]

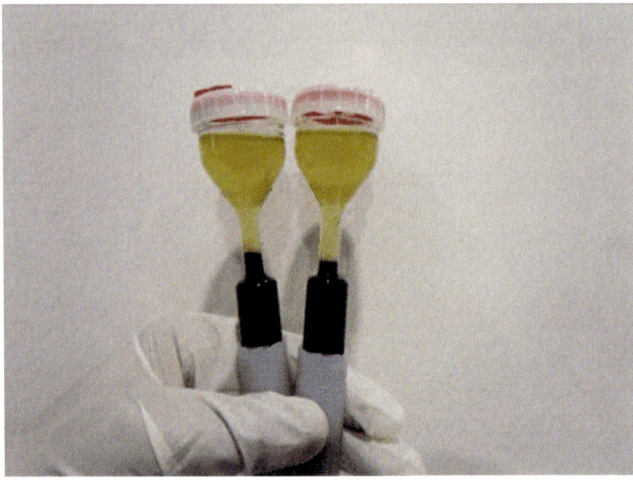

Figure 2: Renew cell kits clearly demonstrate the bottom red blood cell layer, central buffy coat, straw coloured platelet-rich plasma and finally the top layer of platelet-poor plasma harvested with single-spin method in a Remi cold centrifuge at 3,400 rpm and 1,350 relative centrifugal force (RCF) for four minutes.

Anitua et al. used only a single centrifugation spin and collected the volume immediately above the erythrocyte layer. This protocol led to a platelet concentration factor of 2.67 above the baseline value. When all volumes of the upper layer are collected, regardless of whether the buffy coat layer is included, additional spins can be undertaken to achieve higher platelet concentration factors (> 3 times).[20]

Amable et al. performed double centrifugation for platelet isolation, and quantification of cytokines and growth factors on 22 subjects. The best performance for platelet concentration was 300 g for five minutes in the first spin. The second centrifugation of 700 g for 17 minutes was chosen for a lower platelet loss.[21]

Mazzocca et al. analysed three protocols for preparing PRP – a low-speed centrifugation (1,500 rpm for five minutes), a high-speed centrifugation (3,200 rpm for 15 minutes), and double centrifugation with a soft spin of 1,500 rpm for five minutes and a hard spin of 6,300 rpm for 20 minutes. A high platelet concentration with one centrifugation step at 3,200 rpm for 15 minutes was seen compared with the low-speed or double spins.[22]

Gupta et al. compared the manual double-spin method (first spin at 160 g × 10 minutes, second spin at 400 g × 10 minutes) and a commercially available automated device (DrPRP-Kit®, REMI Laboratory Instruments) for PRP preparation. They found that platelet count in both preparations had significantly higher mean platelet count than whole blood ($2.58 \pm 0.81 \times 105/\mu l$, $P < 0.001$). The mean platelet count in manual PRP was statistically significantly higher than in automated PRP. The platelet capture efficiency of the manual method was also statistically significantly higher.[10]

Arshdeep Kumaran adopted a double-spin method of centrifugation: the first spin at 160 g for 10 minutes followed by a second spin at 400 g for 10 minutes at 20°C, to obtain desired platelet concentration of four to seven times the whole blood.[6]

Du et al. studied temperature-controlled PRP (t-PRP), in which exogenous anticoagulants and procoagulants were not used. Ten ml of whole blood was added in 15 ml centrifugation tubes and centrifuged at 200 g for 10 minutes at 4°C. Subsequently, the plasma was transferred to new tubes and centrifuged again at 1,550 for 10 minutes at 4°C. One ml of plasma at the bottom and precipitated platelets was used as t-PRP. The t-PRP was transferred to a new glass tube and then incubated for 15 min at 37°C and then served as activated t-PRP.[23]

Araki et al. obtained a PRP sample having 70–80% recovery of platelets and 10–35% recovery of WBC by application of low accelerations of 70× g for 10 minutes for the first spin.[27] For the second spin, an acceleration of 230× g for 10 minutes was applied. The platelet concentration factor was 7.4 times greater than the baseline after removing about one-tenth of the PPP and adding ethylenediaminetetraacetic acid (EDTA) as an anticoagulant. However, when ACD was used the platelet recovery efficiency was only 35%. This was attributed to the anticoagulant decreasing the platelet integrity in the sample. Therefore, the integrity of platelets is an important parameter that has to be evaluated.[24]

Dhurat et al. found that at 900 g × 5 minutes for the first centrifugation and 1,000 g × 10 minutes for second centrifugation with a temperature of 16°C in a refrigerated centrifuge (Remi CM-8 plus; Remiworld, India), the PRP yield was found to be optimum. Authors consistently recorded platelet counts exceeding 10 lakhs/ml using the mentioned parameters.[12]

Franco et al. obtained a platelet concentration of 8.5 times higher ($603 \times 103/\mu l$) by following the protocol of first centrifugation at 400 g for 10 minutes and 800 g for 10 minutes for the second spin of the buffy coat.[25]

Classification of PRP

Platelet concentrates can be classified into four main families based on their cell content and the architecture of the fibrin.[14]

Pure platelet-rich plasma (P-PRP) or leukocyte-poor platelet-rich plasma preparations are leucocyte poor and have low-density fibrin network on activation. They are used as liquid solutions or as activated gel. After the first slow spin, only the superficial buffy coat layer is aspirated and the second centrifugation is performed; an example is PRGF (plasma-rich in growth factors or preparation-rich in growth factors).

For leukocyte and platelet-rich plasma (L-PRP) products, the entire buffy coat layer and upper 1–2 mm of red blood cell layer are taken out and centrifuged. These are preparations with leukocytes and with the formation of a low-density fibrin network on activation. The majority of the commercial or experimental systems belong to this group.

Pure platelet-rich fibrin (P-PRF) or leukocyte-poor platelet-rich fibrin are leukocyte-poor with a high-density fibrin network, existing only in a strongly activated gel form. Leukocyte and platelet-rich fibrin (L-PRF) are second-generation PRP product preparations with leukocytes and a high-density fibrin network. Blood is centrifuged after collection immediately without any anticoagulant, thrombin or CaC_{l2}.There is the formation of three different layers due to the natural coagulation process – the lowest is the RBC layer, the middle is the L-PRF layer and the top layer is acellular plasma. The PRF clot is pressed between two gauzes to form a strong membrane.

Factors affecting PRP

The platelet yield depends on various parameters such as blood withdrawal technique, temperature, size and shape of the container used, rate and time of spin, anticoagulant used and activation of PRP.[6,12]

Blood withdrawal technique

To avoid unintentional activation of platelets it is better to use large-bore needles (> 22) to draw the blood and re-inject PRP.[26]

Waters and Roberts found that there was a decrease in platelet counts with longer draw time.[27]

Temperature

The optimum temperature for the PRP procedure as stated by Arshdeep Kumaran is between 20 and 22°C. The platelet viability is assured by carrying out the process in a refrigerated centrifuge at 20°C.[6]

According to the Association for the Advancement of Blood & Biotherapies (AABB), manual recommended temperature for centrifugation of blood for obtaining PRP is 21–24°C.[28] Macey et al. also stated that cooling may retard platelet activation, and this may be essential in obtaining PRP with viable platelets.[29] Many authors have used a temperature level of 12–16°C during centrifugation for best platelet recovery.[12]

Although PRP is processed currently at 37 °C or room temperature (RT) – 20–25 °C, low temperatures enhance platelet activation and improve the release of dense and alpha granules.[9] Cold preconditioning increases the release of platelet-derived pro-angiogenic molecules, and promotes the release of growth factors and cytokines by platelets.[30]

Centrifugation

A centrifuge amplifies the effect of gravity by providing centrifugal force which can be many thousand times the force of gravity, thus accelerating the sedimentation.[12]

The separation of cellular constituents of blood is achieved by "differential centrifugation". In differential centrifugation, acceleration force is adjusted leading to sedimentation of certain cellular constituents, and other constituents are left in suspension. The relative centrifugal force or RCF is the force required for the separation of two phases. RCF is expressed as multiples of the earth's gravitational field (g). By accelerating g, speedy sedimentation is achieved. The g-force is the actual force being exerted on the spinning rotor's contents, which further leads to the separation of the aqueous solutions.[14] Revolutions per minute (rpm) are calculated using the following equation:[31] $g = 1.118 \times 10^{-5} \times r \times S^2$ where 'g' is the RCF, R is the radius of the rotor from the centre of the rotor to the sample (cm) and S is the speed of the centrifuge (revolutions per minute).

The RCF calculation is dependent on the radius of the centrifuge rotor used.[12]

Choice of anticoagulant

There will be the formation of a blood clot if no anticoagulant is used, and serum can be obtained but without an increase in the platelet concentration. Coagulation is not intended to occur before the concentration of the platelets; hence, blood must be collected in the presence of anticoagulants.[32]

It is important to choose an anticoagulant that is capable of preserving the platelets' best possible functionality, integrity and morphology.[12]

EDTA (Ethylenediaminetetraacetic acid)

EDTA causes platelet swelling and activation,[33] and may change platelet morphology from a discoid to an irregular spherical shape.[32] It may damage platelet membrane [12] and suppress platelet degranulation.[17] The use of EDTA faces ethical issues, such as being pointed to as a persistent pollutant in natural environments, and there are impediments to its use in certain countries.[32] The mean platelet volume in the EDTA group increases after the centrifugation, which may be an indicator of change in morphology and thus, platelet activation.[32] EDTA-anticoagulation yielded the highest counts of platelets, but platelet recovery was less;[32] EDTA increased RBC counts the most.[33] EDTA suppresses the regenerative activity of cells that are involved in tissue regeneration, e.g. stromal cells.[32]

Anticoagulant citrate dextrose solution A (ACD-A)

ACD and citrate theophylline adenosine dipyridamole (CTAD) are more efficient in maintaining platelet morphology than heparin and sodium citrate.[32] PRP with ACD and CTAD anticoagulants resulted in higher transforming growth factor (TGF)β-1 concentration and induction of mesenchymal stem cell (MSC) proliferation.[32] It was most capable of maintaining intraplatelet signal transduction mechanisms during PRP formulation.[32] If ACD is used, the reduction of the tube size may increase platelet recovery.[32]

ACD-A preserves platelet morphology (size) and functionality (activation and growth factor retention) better than other anticoagulants.[33] It has a lower chelating ability compared with EDTA and has no detectable adverse effects on platelets, leukocytes or other cells involved in tissue regeneration.[33] ACD-A) is preferred and best supports platelet viability; the citrate binds calcium to create anticoagulation. The dextrose, buffers and other ingredients support the metabolic needs of platelets.[7] ACD binds calcium and prevents the clotting cascade initiation by the coagulation proteins. Citrate also makes blood more acidic than its physiological pH. As some growth factors are influenced by the tissue pH, some protocols recommend that PRP should be buffered back to a physiologic range before injection.[17]

Sodium citrate

Sodium citrate at 3.8% has a pH of 7.8 whereas ACD-A has a pH of 4.9. In addition, 3.8% sodium citrate contains 24.4 mg of citrate ion/ml whereas the citrate ion concentration in ACD-A is 15.6 mg/ml. In several species, the alterations in the pH and extracellular iCa concentration of PRP can affect platelet aggregation in vitro, with aggregation typically impaired at acidic pH and lower extracellular iCa concentrations.[12]

Citrate phosphate dextrose (CPD)

CPD is similar to ACD-A but has fewer supportive ingredients so is 10% less effective in maintaining the platelet viability.[7]

Heparin

Heparin is inappropriate for the preparation of PRP due to the difficulties that are inherent in the quality control and retrieval of coagulation activity. Heparin induces platelet aggregation and adhesion to WBC; hence, platelet counts cannot necessarily be accurately determined by the automated haematology analyser.[33]

Activation of platelets

The term "activation" refers to two key processes: (1) degranulation of platelets to release growth factors from α-granules, and (2) fibrinogen cleavage to initiate matrix/fibrin network formation, a clotting process that allows the formation of a platelet gel and therefore confines the secretion of molecules to the chosen site.[33] If PRP is activated too strongly, there will be the formation of a bivalent, unstable fibrin network. If it is activated in a more physiologic manner, there will be the formation of a tetramolecular stable network that enhances cells and growth factor enmeshment. It is undesirable to have overly viscous PRP when injecting into the soft tissue.[14]

The most commonly used activation methods are $CaCl_2$, autologous thrombin, their combination, mechanical trauma, and/or collagen type I to mimic the clinical conditions where their presence in the treated connective tissues should induce an in situ or spontaneous platelet activation. The latter is currently chosen for several PRP applications since it is considered to be an easier and more effective strategy to deliver platelet bioactive molecules.[34]

Recent evidence suggests that non-activated or resting PRP may be injected, and slow spontaneous platelet activation occurs due to exposure to dermal collagen and thrombin.[4]

A direct PRP activation in situ might overcome some of the shortcomings related to the use of thrombin, resulting in the risk of potentially life-threatening coagulopathies, and CaC_{12}, which is sometimes associated with a burning sensation due to low pH;[34] xenogeneic thrombin may trigger immunogenic reactions.[23] Newer activation methods including usage of Triton X and sonication have also been found to be effective.[35]

Thawing frozen platelets as a mechanical method activates growth factors from platelets therefore further activation is not necessary.[35]

Patient factors

Patient factors also play a role in platelet concentration. Fasting patients had lower concentrations than those who ate a high-fat meal. The timings of venepuncture can also affect concentration, with the optimal time being in the afternoon.[17]

Physiological differences between individuals such as haematocrit variability and size of platelets may lead to inter-individual variability. Intra-individual variation of 19.7% (range 0.5–56.3%) in the platelet counts obtained by the same method on four different occasions 15 days apart has also been reported.[10]

Spin rates

Lower spin rates had higher platelet yields, which led to the hypothesis that high rates could cause platelet clumping or disintegration.[17] The greater the distance from the axis of the centrifugal rotor, the greater the centrifugal force acting on the particle. The mean centrifugal force applied to the erythrocytes decreased with the smaller mean distance from the rotor for the two samples of blood processed under the same angular velocity.[18,36]

Effect of time on centrifugation

Longer time periods slightly increased platelet recovery and decreased the concentrations of WBC in the upper layer. Therefore, time could be a control parameter when low levels of WBC, such as granulocytes and lymphocytes, are required in the PRP sample.[18]

Effects of the processed volume

The processing of a larger volume of whole blood in a single tube decreased the recovery efficiency of platelets and packing of the erythrocytes compared to a smaller volume of WB processed under the same conditions.[18]

Similar results were obtained when different volumes of the upper layer were transferred to the second spin. The concentration of platelets was favoured and the percentage of remaining platelets in the PPP decreased for the smaller volumes processed.[18]

Presence of WBCs

Currently, there is disagreement over whether the presence of WBCs[4,18] in PRP provides any benefit. Authors who are in favour of the presence of WBCs advocate that the presence of leukocytes provides protection from infection, increases growth factor release and contributes to angiogenesis, matrix production and hypercellularity.

On the contrary, many researchers do not recommend the presence of WBCs in PRP. Neutrophils may release reactive oxygen species and pro-inflammatory cytokines, which may increase inflammation and destroy surrounding tissue. They may also increase matrix metalloproteinase levels, which can cause degradation of the matrix. WBC concentration is directly correlated to catabolic gene expression which may impair tissue healing.

Presence of RBCs

Erythrocytes may represent a source of released reactive oxygen species and might act as an inflammatory stress inducer.[4]

Utility of platelet aggregation inhibitor

Anticoagulants do not interrupt the aggregation of platelets. This has been overlooked in preparing PRP conventionally. Aggregated platelets stick to the syringe wall and do not get easily detached from them. As the primary aggregation of platelets is reversible, the platelets come off from the wall and float in the plasma again after several hours. Waiting for such a long time is not feasible in daily practice. Therefore, a platelet aggregation inhibitor (PGE1) can be used to prevent this aggregation.[37]

Helpful tips for PRP procedure standardization[12]

1. Donor percentage haematocrit (the ratio of the volume of RBCs to the total volume of blood) is relevant for plasma yield optimization. Blood with a low haematocrit percentage has more plasma available, thereby diluting the concentration of platelets in plasma.
2. Blood samples collected in ACD tubes should be inverted 5–10 times so there is proper mixing of the anticoagulant and blood. If mixing is not done small fibrin clots may form, causing a falsely decreased platelet count.
3. After the first spin, if a large plasma volume is obtained, then it would need a higher 'g' to concentrate platelets at the bottom of the tube (law of velocity).
4. PRP should be separated from the PPP soon after centrifugation because the concentrated platelets slowly diffuse into the PPP over time and would reduce the platelet count of the PRP preparation.
5. For counting of the platelets in final PRP concentrate, it must be re-suspended for at least 5–10 minutes to allow equal distribution of platelets before counting.

PRP should be kept in small diameter tubes with caps (to minimize surface area to atmosphere) as the pH can increase by diffusion of CO_2 out of the plasma, thus potentially causing spontaneous aggregation.[38]

Future directions: newer forms of PRP and bio filler

Newer forms of platelet-rich plasma (PRP) are the following:[39]

1. APRF – advanced monocyte-rich PRF
2. IPRF – injectable PRF
3. CGF – concentrated growth factors
4. HAS – hyperacute serum
5. TPRF – titanium activated PRF

Preparation of iPRF

Blood is centrifuged at low speeds (60 g for 3 minutes) without anticoagulant in special plastic tubes slowing down the clotting process. Liquid PRF solution is formed which takes 15–20 minutes to clot. PRF produces more cumulative growth factors than PRP and releases them in a more controlled way. Platelet concentration amplification is much lower than PRP.[39]

Bio filler

Platelet-poor plasma-based bio filler is an innovative and economical alternative to expensive hyaluronic acid-based fillers.[40,41] It is easy to obtain and autologous. Ten ml of patient's blood mixed with 1 ml anticoagulant acid citrate dextrose is centrifuged at 3,200 RPM for 8 minutes. The plasma fraction is withdrawn and again centrifuged at 1,000 RPM for five minutes. The upper part i.e. PPP (platelet-poor plasma) of approximately 4.5 ml is taken in a 5 ml syringe. Calcium gluconate in the proportion of 0.01 ml per 1 ml of PPP is added. This is incubated in hot water at 100°C for five minutes and then in cold water with an initial temperature of 7°C, and later increased to 10°C for five minutes; 3 ml of viscous gel as bio filler is formed.[40] The gel has a direct volumetric filling effect due to denatured gelled proteins and fibrin bundles, which provide constant stability and volume.[40]

Conclusion

PRP continues to evolve as an important treatment modality with multiple applications in dermatology. There is the presence of a wide range of preparation protocols, devices and centrifuges for varying indications leading to the formation of a number of different platelet concentrates, and all of them are categorized as PRP.

In this chapter, we aimed to optimize current PRP preparation protocols to standardize the PRP preparation method.

References

1. Alser OH, Goutos I. The evidence behind the use of platelet-rich plasma (PRP) in scar management: a literature review. *Scars Burn Heal*. 2018 Nov 18;**4**:2059513118808773.
doi: 10.1177/2059513118808773.
PMID: 30479843; PMCID: PMC6243404.
2. Garg S, Manchanda S. Platelet-rich plasma – an "elixir" for treatment of alopecia: personal experience on 117 patients with review of literature. *Stem Cell Investig*. 2017;**4**:64. doi:10.21037/sci.2017.06.07.

3. Marx RE. Platelet-rich plasma: evidence to support its use. *J Oral Maxillofac Surg*. 2004; **62**: 489-496. ISSN 0278-2391, https://doi.org/10.1016/j.joms.2003.12.003.
4. Stevens J, Khetarpal S. Platelet-rich plasma for androgenetic alopecia: a review of the literature and proposed treatment protocol. *Int J Women's Dermatology*. 2019;**5**:46-51. ISSN 2352-6475, https://doi.org/10.1016/j.ijwd.2018.08.004.
5. Lana JFSD, Vicente EF, Weglein A, Belangero WD, Assis FD, Mansano AM. Platelet-rich plasma in pain medicine. In: Maffulli N, editor. Platelet rich plasma in musculoskeletal practice. London: Springer-Verlag; 2016. p. 32. doi: 10.1007/978-1-4471-7271-0.
6. Arshdeep Kumaran MS. Platelet-rich plasma in dermatology: boon or a bane? *Indian J Dermatol Venereol Leprol*. 2014;**80**:5-14.
7. Marx RE. DDS platelet-rich plasma (PRP): what is PRP and what is not PRP? *Implant Dent*. 2001;**10**:225-228.
8. Arora NS, Ramanayake S, Ren Y-F, Romanos, GE. Platelet-rich plasma: a literature review. *Implant Dent*. 2009;**18:**303-310 doi: 10.1097/ID.0b013e31819e8ec6
9. Rughetti A, Giusti I, D'Ascenzo S, Leocata P, Carta G, Pavan A, et al. Platelet gel-released supernatant modulates the angiogenic capability of human endothelial cells. *Blood Transfus*. 2008;**6**:12-7.
10. Gupta V, Parihar AS, Pathak M, Sharma VK. Comparison of platelet-rich plasma prepared using two methods: manual double spin method versus a commercially available automated device. *Indian Dermatol Online J*. 2020;**11**:575-579. doi: 10.4103/idoj.idoj_653_19.
11. Gentile P, Garcovich S, Bielli A, Scioli MG, Orlandi A, Cervelli V. The effect of platelet-rich plasma in hair regrowth: a randomized placebo-controlled trial. *Stem Cells Transl Med*. 2015;**4**:1317-1323.
12. Dhurat R, Sukesh M. Principles and methods of preparation of platelet-rich plasma: a review and author's perspective. *J Cutan Aesthet Surg*. 2014;**7**:189-197. doi:10.4103/0974-2077.150734.
13. American Association of Blood Banks technical manual committee. Method 6.11: Preparation of platelets from whole blood. In: Vengelen-Tyler V, editor. AABB Technical Manual, 13th ed. Bethesda (MD): American Association of Blood Banks; 1999. p. 725.
14. Garg S, Manchanda S, Garg C. The wonder tool platelet rich plasma in cosmetic dermatology, trichology and hair transplant, dermatologic surgery and procedures. In: Vereecken P, editor. Dermatologic Surgery and Procedures. IntechOpen [Internet] February 2018. doi: 10.5772/intechopen.70287.

https://www.intechopen.com/books/dermatologic-surgery-and-procedures/the-wonder-tool-platelet-rich-plasma-in-cosmetic-dermatology-trichology-and-hair-transplant

15. Fukaya M, Ito A. A new economic method for preparing platelet-rich plasma. *Plast Reconstr Surg Glob Open*. 2014;**2**:e162. doi:10.1097/GOX.0000000000000109
16. Kakudo N, Kushida S, Kusumoto, K. Platelet-rich plasma: the importance of platelet separation and concentration, plastic and reconstructive surgery. March;123:1135-1136 doi: 10.1097/PRS.0b013e31819a3575
17. Collins T, Alexander D, Barkatali B. Platelet-rich plasma: a narrative review. *EFORT Open Rev*. 2021 Apr;**6**:225-235. doi: 10.1302/2058-5241.6.200017.
18. Perez AGM, Lana JFSD, Rodrigues AA, Luzo ACM, Belangero WD, Santana MHA. Relevant aspects of centrifugation step in the preparation of platelet-rich plasma. *ISRN Hematol*. 2014;**2014**:176060. doi: 10.1155/2014/176060.
19. Arora S, Doda V, Kotwal U, Dogra M. Quantification of platelets and platelet derived growth factors from platelet-rich-plasma (PRP) prepared at different centrifugal force (g) and time. *Transfus Apher Sci* 2016;**54**:103–110.
20. Anitua E, Aguirre JJ, Algorta J, Ayerdi E, Cabezas AI, Orive G, et al. Effectiveness of autologous preparation rich in growth factors for the treatment of chronic cutaneous ulcers. *J Biomed Mater Res B Appl Biomater*. 2008 Feb;**84**:415-21.
21. Amable PR, Carias RB, Teixeira MV, da Cruz Pacheco I, Corrêa do Amaral RJ, Granjeiro JM, et al. Platelet-rich plasma preparation for regenerative medicine: Optimization and quantification of cytokines and growth factors. *Stem Cell Res Ther*. 2013;**4**:67.
22. Mazzocca AD, McCarthy MB, Chowaniec DM, Cote MP, Romeo AA, Bradley JP, et al. Platelet-rich plasma differs according to preparation method and human variability. *J Bone Joint Surg Am*. 2012;**94**:308–16.
23. Du L, Miao Y, Li X, Shi P, Hu Z. A novel and convenient method for the preparation and activation of PRP without any additives: temperature controlled PRP. *Biomed Res Int*. 2018; 1761865. https://doi.org/10.1155/2018/1761865
24. Araki J, Jona M, Eto H, Aoi N, Kato H, Suga H, et al. Optimized preparation method of platelet-concentrated plasma and noncoagulating platelet-derived factor concentrates: maximization of platelet concentration and removal of fibrinogen. *Tissue Eng Part C Methods*. 2012;**18**:176–85.

25. Franco D, Franco T, Schettino AM, Filho JM, Vendramin FS. Protocol for obtaining platelet-rich plasma (PRP), platelet-poor plasma (PPP), and thrombin for autologous use. *Aesthetic Plast Surg* 2012;**36**:1254-1259.
26. Harmon K, Hanson R, Bowen J, Greenberg S, Magaziner E, Vandenbosch J, et al. Guidelines for the use of platelet rich plasma. *The International Cellular Medical Society (ICMS)*. 2011. Version 1.0. [updated 2011; cited 23 March 2016] [Internet]. http://www.cellmedicinesociety.org/attachments/370_Section%2010%20-%20Platelet%20Rich%20Plasma%20(PRP)%20Guidelines.pdf
27. Waters JH, Roberts KC. Database review of possible factors influencing point-of-care platelet gel manufacture. *J Extra Corpor Technol*. 2004;**36**:250-254.
28. Sweeny J, Grossman BJ. Blood collection, storage and component preparation methods. In: Brecher M, editor. Technical Manual. 14th ed. Bethesda, MD: American Association of Blood Banks (AABB); 2002. pp. 955-958
29. Macey M, Azam U, McCarthy D, Webb L, Chapman ES, Okrongly D, et al. Evaluation of the anticoagulants EDTA and citrate, theophylline, adenosine, and dipyridamole (CTAD) for assessing platelet activation on the ADVIA 120 hematology system. *Clin Chem*. 2002;48:891-899.
30. Etulain J, Mena HA, Meiss RP, Frechtel G, Gutt S, Negrotto S, et al. An optimised protocol for platelet-rich plasma preparation to improve its angiogenic and regenerative properties. *Sci Rep*. 2018;**8**:1513. https://doi.org/10.1038/s41598-018-19419-6
31. Jain SK, Soni V. Bentley's textbook of pharmaceutics – an adaptation. India: Elsevier India; 2014. pp. 556-565.
32. do Amaral RJFC, da Silva NP, Haddad NF, Lopes LS, Ferreira FD, Filho RB, et al. Platelet-rich plasma obtained with different anticoagulants and their effect on platelet numbers and mesenchymal stromal cells behavior in vitro. *Stem Cells Int*. 2016;2016:7414036. doi:10.1155/2016/7414036.
33. Aizawa H, Kawabata H, Sato A, Masuli H, Watanabe T, Tsujino T, et al. A comparative study of the effects of anticoagulants on pure platelet-rich plasma quality and potency. *Biomedicines*. 2020;**8**:42. doi:10.3390/biomedicines8030042.
34. Cavallo C, Roffi A, Grigolo B, Mariani E, Pratelli L, Merli G, et al. Platelet-rich plasma: the choice of activation method affects the release of bioactive molecules. *Biomed Res Int*. **2016**:2016:6591717. https://doi.org/10.1155/2016/6591717

35. Kim JI, Bae HC, Park HJ, Lee MC, Han HS. Effect of storage conditions and activation on growth factor concentration in platelet-rich plasma. *J. Orthop. Res*. 2020;**38**:777-784. https://doi.org/10.1002/jor.24520
36. Xu J, Gou L, Zhang P, Li H, Qiu S. Platelet-rich plasma and regenerative dentistry. *Aust Dent J.* 2020;**65**:131-142. https://doi.org/10.1111/adj.12754
37. Fukaya M, Ito A. A new economic method for preparing platelet-rich plasma. *Plast Reconstr Surg – Glob Open*. 2014;**2**:e162.
38. Arora S, Agnihotri N. Platelet derived biomaterials for therapeutic use: review of technical aspects. *Indian J Hematol Blood Transfus.* 2017;**33**:159–167.
39. Sharma A, Chouhan K, Bhatia S, Dashore S. Platelet-rich plasma in androgenetic alopecia. *Indian Dermatol Online J.* 2021 Nov 25;**12** (Suppl. 1):S31-S40. doi: 10.4103/idoj.idoj_328_21. PMID: 34976879; PMCID: PMC8664169.
40. Gupta S, Borde Bisht P, Kannan C. Bio-filler: an effective facial rejuvenation tool easy on pocket. *J Cutan Aesthet Surg*. 2020 Jul-Sep;**13**:243-246. doi: 10.4103/JCAS.JCAS_172_19. PMID: 33209005; PMCID: PMC7646418.
41. Dashore S, Dashore A. Platelet poor plasma based biofiller: an innovative alternative to expensive hyaluronic acid based fillers for treatment of chicken pox scars. *J Am Acad Dermatol*. 2021;**84**:e11-e13.

CHAPTER 3

HARVESTING OF PLATELET-RICH PLASMA: SINGLE SPIN VS DOUBLE SPIN

SUJANA LAKKIREDDYGARI, ANUVA BANSAL, SURUCHI GARG

Platelet-rich plasma (PRP) is a novel technique among cell and tissue-based therapies which have gained widespread popularity for a diverse set of indications, across the fields of regenerative medicine and surgery.[1] PRP consists of plasma with a concentration of platelets, which on degranulation release several growth factors (GFs) and cytokines that function to enhance cell proliferation, differentiation and angiogenesis, thus augmenting the natural repair mechanisms. In the authors' opinion, PRP may be termed a *dermabiologic*, a new emerging treatment modality in the ever-evolving segment of modern healthcare, known as *autologous biologics*.

Harvesting of PRP

Despite the advancement and the popularity of PRP, the lack of a standardized preparation protocol precludes the comparison of the results obtained from various studies.[2] In the recent past, a number of commercially available kits and personalized protocols have been used, which differ significantly in terms of the volume of blood, the target platelet count and the type of activator used, underlining the need for the development of a uniform PRP preparation technique.

Factors affecting PRP[3]

A number of factors are currently known to influence the yield of PRP and include:

- characteristics of the centrifugation device
- "g" (gravitational) force applied during the centrifugation process
- temperature
- volume of blood collected
- anticoagulation method
- duration of each spin cycle
- number of spin cycles
- method of separation into serum, cells and platelet fraction.

Authors have hypothesized that the shape of the PRP kit and the adequate maintenance of temperature during the centrifugation process also significantly affects the target platelet count achieved and the overall outcome of the procedure.

Characteristics of the centrifugation device

Over time, the earth's gravitational force (g-force) is sufficient to separate various types of particles. A tube containing whole blood and an anticoagulant will eventually separate into plasma, red blood cells and white blood cell fractions, when left undisturbed for sufficient time. However, the length of time required for such a separation prevents its practical application in a real-life scenario. Moreover, a faster separation technique will prevent the natural degradation of biological products which also happens over time.

In clinical practice, centrifugation allows for a faster means for separation of the blood components. The rate of separation of the particles depends on the centrifugal g-force which is influenced by the particle size and density. Highly dense or large particles travel faster and become separated from less dense or smaller particles. Settling or sedimentation of particles is explained by the Stokes equation, which describes the movement of a sphere in a "g" field.[1]

The Stokes equation

$$v = \frac{d^2(p - L)Xg}{18n}$$

Where:

v = velocity of the particle (sphere), or sedimentation rate or velocity of sedimentation

d = diameter

p = density of the particle

L = density of the medium
g = gravitational force
n = medium viscosity

From the equation it can be concluded that the sedimentation rate increases with an increase in the size of the particle, the density of the medium, the g-force and with a decrease in the viscosity of the medium.

However, the g-force is not enough to separate the tiny particles (e.g. platelets); hence, centrifugation has been developed, which increases the g-force by producing a centrifugal force (a spinning force around an axis). The main principle of centrifugation is Stokes' law.[4,5]

When a centrifugal force is applied to whole blood, leukocytes and erythrocytes will settle faster in plasma than the platelets and will become separated.[6] The centrifugal forces are different due to a difference in the radius, density and viscosity of cellular particles.[7] Hence, the sedimentation rates of platelets, erythrocytes and leukocytes also vary, and this key principle underlies PRP preparation. These parameters also influence the final composition of the PRP obtained.

There are many different types of centrifuges but the most commonly used are the fixed-angle centrifuges. The centrifugation data is stated in units of gravity (g), or relative centrifugal force (RCF) which is shown via rotations per minute (rpm).[8] The present-day centrifuge machines can automatically convert the values from RCF to rpm and vice versa. RCF is calculated as follows:

$$RCF=\frac{r\omega 2}{g}$$

or

$$RCF=11.18 x r x \left(\frac{n}{1000}\right)2$$

r = radius from the central axis in centimetres
ω = angular velocity per unit time during centrifugation
g = Earth's gravitational force
n = rotational speed in rpm

During centrifugation, as the radius from the central axis increases the RCF also increases, thus amplifying the sedimentation of particles. First to sediment are the erythrocytes, which occupy the lowermost part of the tube, and the next layer above this is the buffy coat layer, composed of leukocytes and platelets. Above this layer lies the PRP or the platelet concentrate, and over this the platelet-poor plasma layer is present.

The authors use the Ycellbio or Renewcell PRP kit for centrifugation during PRP preparation. As previously described, the shape of the centrifuge tube positively affects the yield, and the narrowing of the tube at the centre, as present in this kit, increases the r value as well as the RCF, resulting in increased sedimentation and an effective concentration of platelets. The shape of the PRP kit may also optimize the centrifugation parameters, by decreasing the number of spins and the time required to achieve the target platelet concentration.

The "g" (gravitational) force during centrifugation

The force exerted during centrifugation affects the kinetics and influences the number of growth factors released from the platelets. Amable et al. observed the impact of the variations in force and temperature during centrifugation, on the release of growth factors after activation, and reported that the optimization of RCF, time and temperature influenced the final platelet yield and purity.[9] Moreover, an increase in temperature and a decrease in plasma density was found to affect the blood cell behaviour under the same centrifugation conditions. Thus, longer centrifugation spins would be better applied with a lower RCF, ensuring that the platelets are still isolated in the upper fraction.[9]

A force of 3,800 rpm (3,731 × g) for a period of 4 minutes has been deemed to be the optimal condition to yield the highest platelet concentration of 8.3×10^{10} platelets in 245 ml of plasma, from 478 ml of whole blood, as determined by Kahn et al.[10]

A faster centrifugation without refrigeration can generate a significant amount of heat which could lead to the premature activation of platelets, precipitating an untimely release of growth factors.

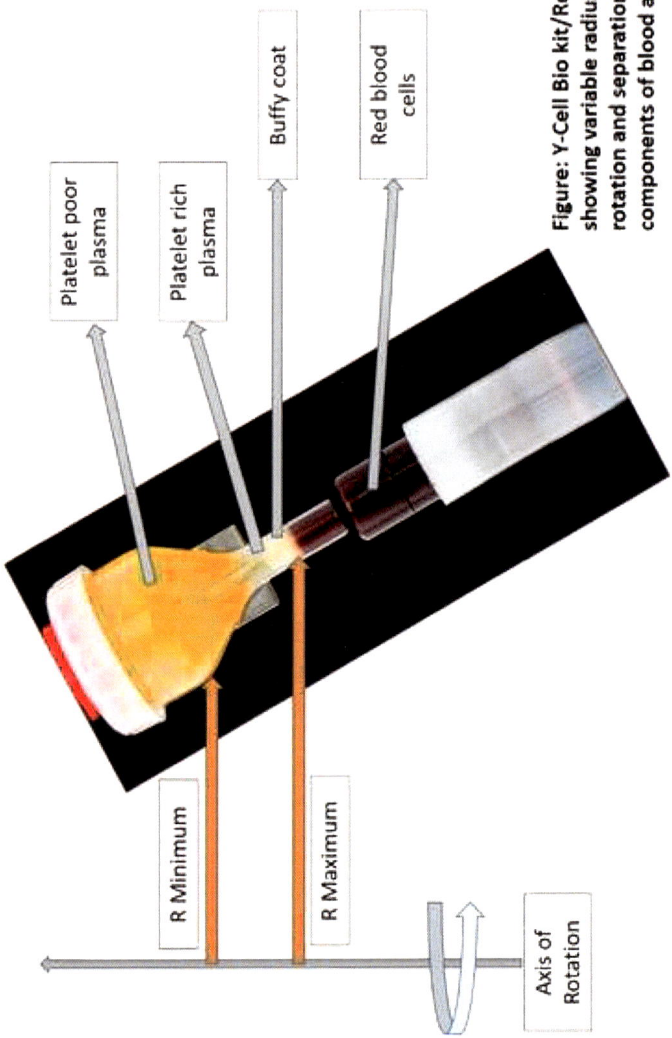

Figure: Y-Cell Bio kit/Renew cell kit showing variable radius from axis of rotation and separation of different components of blood after centrifugation

The authors suggest using an optimal force of 1350 with 3400 rpm for 4 minutes at 12°C for effective platelet capture.

Temperature

Enzymatic activity, as well as protein stability, are heat-sensitive and temperature-dependent processes. As previously outlined, heat production during centrifugation may cause protein or enzymatic denaturation as well as a premature, untimely activation of platelets and subsequent release of growth factors.[11] PRP preparation requires adequate temperature maintenance which can be achieved via a refrigerated centrifuge at 12–16°C

Amable et al.[9] prepared PRP using a refrigerated centrifuge maintaining a temperature of 8°C to 16°C, which resulted in a good platelet yield. Platelet activation can be delayed with cooling, and some authors suggest an ideal temperature of 8°C to retard platelet stimulation.[12]

Sample volume

Sample volume tends to vary depending upon the surface area and location affected. Most studies recommend injecting an amount of approximately 0.1 ml to 0.4 ml per cm^2, injected 1 cm apart.[13] Variations in the amount injected exist and Alves et al. used 0.15 ml in a 1×1 cm^2 area over the scalp with good results, while Gentile et al. used 0.1 ml/cm^2 as interfollicular injections with a 30G needle, and achieved a comparable outcome.[14,15]

Anticoagulation method

Anticoagulants prevent the clotting of blood, which starts right from the time that the blood is drawn.[16] Several anticoagulants are commonly used including citrate, ethylenediaminetetraacetic acid (EDTA), heparin oxalates and sodium fluoride. The appropriate choice for an anticoagulant is the one that best preserves the integrity and function of platelets. The most commonly used ones are acid citrate and EDTA. However, as EDTA may cause damage to the platelet membrane, its use is not routinely advocated. Therefore, the most common choice for an anticoagulant, utilized in several studies, is acid citrate dextrose-A.[16]

Duration and number of spin cycles

The majority of the studies on PRP utilize a double-spin technique and very few studies are endorsing a single-spin methodology. The authors hypothesize that, by changing the shape of the PRP kit, the number of spins and duration can be reduced with effective PRP capture. The authors have used a single spin for 4 minutes with a good platelet yield (three times the baseline concentration). Anitua et al. captured enriched PRP with a single spin.[2] Alves et al. found a three-fold increase in platelets above the baseline with a single spin.[14] Kahn et al. obtained an eight-fold increase in platelets above the baseline with a single spin for 4 minutes at 3,731 RCF.[10]

Activation of PRP

A controversy exists regarding the activation of PRP prior to injecting it. Although the most common activators used are mechanical trauma, calcium chloride, calcium gluconate, thrombin and collagen, it has been suggested that if PRP is used in soft tissue, no need for activation exists as collagen acts as a natural activator. Furthermore, initiation of inflammation at the target area after PRP injection favours its activation, precluding the need for exogenous activation.[1]

PRP yield

Richness of PRP yield can be ascertained based on the increase in the concentration of platelets compared to the baseline. Most of the studies consider an average of a 5- to 8-fold increase in the baseline platelet count as an effective PRP concentrate. Calculation of platelet collection efficiency and platelet enrichment factor has been elucidated below.[17,18]

$$\text{Platelet collection efficiency} = \frac{\text{volume of prp(ml)} \times \text{platelet count of prp/ml}}{\text{volume of blood sample(ml)} \times \text{platelet count of blood sample/ml}} \times 100$$

$$\text{Platelet enrichment factor(fold)} = \frac{\text{Platelet concentration of PRP}}{\text{Platelet concentration of whole blood}}$$

In a blood sample, 6% cells are platelets, 93% are RBCs and 1% cells are white blood cells. The goal of PRP is to enrich the platelets through centrifugation, and *reverse the platelet to RBC ratio* to achieve a 94% concentration of platelets and a 5% concentration of RBCs.[19] Current literature suggests that effective tissue regeneration requires a platelet concentration of at least 1 million platelets/μl or five times the baseline concentration.[20] Platelets are a storehouse of several growth factors (GFs), which act on cells such as epithelial, endothelial and stem cells, fibroblasts and osteoblasts, and are responsible for the therapeutic benefits of PRP.[19] The secretion of these GFs begins 10 minutes after platelet activation and more than 95% of the secretion is completed within 1 hour, thus warranting the application of PRP within 10 minutes of clot initiation.[16]

A 1:10 ratio of PRP to whole blood must be obtained for standardization of PRP. Vascular remodelling begins at a platelet concentration of 1.5×10^6 platelets/ml, also called the magic number, and concentrations higher or lower than this are considered detrimental to the process of angiogenesis. Recent evidence indicates that a platelet count of 1 million/ml is essential for the enhancement of wound repair and regeneration, and may be considered the working definition for therapeutic PRP.[16]

With the advent of the newer generations of PRP such as iPRF (injectable PRF), aPRF (advanced PRF), the concept of a higher concentration of platelets or attaining a magic number has become controversial.[21] These are less concentrated platelet preparations that are giving good results, according to upcoming literature, but we need to perform head-to-head comparative studies to elucidate the ideal concentration of platelets. This should show whether exhaustive double-spin methods should actually be required in the future to attain so-called magic numbers, or that three to four times the concentration of platelets from baseline would be sufficient to attain the desired results. After all, the out-of-body time increases considerably in the double-spin method and it may temper platelet morphology, which ideally should be studied under electron microscopy.

The roles of various growth factors released from platelets are shown in Table 1.[22]

Table 1: Role of various growth factors released from platelets in PRP

Growth Factors	Actions
PDGF αα, αβ, ββ	Mitogenic for fibroblasts, endothelial cells and smooth muscles. Chemotactic for fibroblasts and macrophages.
TGF β_1, β_2	Mitogenic for fibroblasts and smooth muscles. Chemotactic for fibroblasts, macrophages and keratinocytes. Mediates angiogenesis. Inhibits endothelial cells, keratinocytes and lymphocytes. Regulates the matrix proteins and collagen, fibronectin, proteoglycans and matrix-degrading proteins.
EGF	Mitogenic for fibroblasts, endothelial cells and keratinocytes. Mediates angiogenesis.
HGF	Mediates regeneration.
FGF	Mediates regeneration and tissue organization.
FGF-9	Helps in the generation of new follicles.
VEGF	Mediates angiogenesis. Mitogenic and chemotactic for endothelial cells.

PDGF = platelet-derived growth factor, TGF = transforming growth factor, EGF = epidermal growth factor, HGF = hepatocyte growth factor, FGF = fibroblast growth factor, VEGF = vascular endothelial growth factor.

Level of injection

The level should be intradermal or subdermal injections in serial puncture techniques for skin rejuvenation, and deep in the level of scar for scar remodelling. Over the scalp these injections are given interfollicular, ideally parallel to the direction of hair and can be placed 0.5 to 1 cm apart.

PRP extraction (steps followed by the authors)

Depending on the target area of application, the amount of whole blood required is usually collected from the cubital vein. As a protocol, a 13 ml sample is collected for the face and 26 ml for the scalp.

1. Venous blood (13 ml) is collected into the Ycellbio PRP kit/Renewcell kit which contains 1.5 ml of acid citrate dextrose-A (ACD-A) and is centrifuged at 3,400 rpm and 1,350 relative centrifugal force (RCF) for a period of 4 minutes at 12°C.
2. With a large-bore 18 G needle, the PRP fraction along with the upper two-thirds of the buffy coat layer is pipetted out (nearly 1.5–2 ml).
3. Without using an activator, PRP is injected intradermally into the face and at the interfollicular level into the scalp, trauma activating as the spontaneous activator for the degranulation of platelets.

Conclusion

The authors present a simple PRP protocol that is safe and ensures a good platelet yield to provide consistent and uniform results. We personally recommend using a standardized, easily reproducible protocol for all indications using a single-spin technique with an hourglass tube, which provides good platelet capture. Great variation exists in the technique of PRP preparation and currently, there is no consensus regarding a standardized treatment protocol, highlighting the importance of a good number of studies with larger sample sizes to establish a validated, uniform technique.

References

1. Schiavone G, Raskovic D, Greco J, Abeni D. Platelet-rich plasma for androgenetic alopecia: a pilot study. *Dermatol Surg*. 2014 Sep;**40**:1010-9.

2. Anitua E, Pino A, Martinez N, Orive G, Berridi D. The effect of plasma rich in growth factors on pattern hair loss: a pilot study. *Dermatol Surg.* 2017 May;**43**:658-670.
3. Chahla J, Cinque ME, Piuzzi NS, Mannava S, Geeslin AG, Murray IR, et al. A call for standardization in platelet-rich plasma preparation protocols and composition reporting: A systematic review of the clinical orthopaedic literature. *J Bone Joint Surg Am.* 2017 Oct 18;**99**:1769-79.
4. Yin W, Xu Z, Sheng J, Xie X, Zhang C. Erythrocyte sedimentation rate and fibrinogen concentration of whole blood influences the cellular composition of platelet-rich plasma obtained from centrifugation methods. *Exp Ther Med* 2017;**14**:1909-18.
5. Yin W, Xu H, Sheng J, Zhu Z, Jin D, Hsu P, et al. Optimization of pure platelet rich plasma preparation: A comparative study of pure platelet rich plasma obtained using different centrifugal conditions in a single donor model. *Exp Ther Med* 2017 Sep;**14**:2060-70.
6. Arnoczky SP, Sheibani-Rad S. The basic science of platelet-rich plasma (PRP): what clinicians need to know. *Sports Med Arthrosc Rev.* 2013 Dec;**214**:180-5.
7. Araki J, Jona M, Eto H, Aoi N, Kato H, Suga H, et al. Optimized preparation method of platelet-concentrated plasma and noncoagulating platelet-derived factor concentrates: Maximization of platelet concentration and removal of fibrinogen. *Tissue Eng Part C Methods* 2012;**18**:176–85.
8. Pendleton M. Descriptions of melissopalynological methods involving centrifugation should include data for calculating relative centrifugal force (RCF) or should express data in units of RCF or gravities (g). *Grana* 2006;**45**:71-2.
9. Amable PR, Carias RB, Teixeira MV, da Cruz Pacheco I, Corrêa do Amaral RJ, Granjeiro JM, et al. Platelet-rich plasma preparation for regenerative medicine: Optimization and quantification of cytokines and growth factors. *Stem Cell Res Ther.* 2013;**4**:67.
10. Kahn RA, Cossette I, Friedman LI. Optimum centrifugation conditions for the preparation of platelet and plasma products. *Transfusion* 1976;**16**:162–5.
11 Tuck MK, Chan DW, Chia D, Godwin AK, Grizzle WE, Krueger KE, et al. Standard operating operating procedures for serum and plasma collection: early detection research network network consensus statement standard operating procedure integration working group. *J Proteome Res.* 2009 Jan;**8**:113-7.

12. Macey M, Azam U, McCarthy D, Webb L, Chapman ES, Okrongly D et al. Evaluation of the anticoagulants EDTA and citrate, theophylline, adenosine, and dipyridamole (CTAD) for assessing platelet activation on the ADVIA 120 hematology system. *Clin Chem*. 2002 Jun;**48**:891-9.
13. Schiavone G, Roskovic D, Greco J, Abeni D. Platelet-rich plasma for Androgenetic alopecia: a pilot study. *Dermatol Surg.* 2014 Sep;**40**:1010-19.
14. Alves R, Grimalt R. Randomized placebo-controlled, double-blind, half-head study to assess the efficacy of platelet-rich plasma on the treatment of androgenetic alopecia. *Dermatol Surg.* 2016 Apr;**42**:491-7.
15. Gentile P, Garcovich S, Bielli A, Scioli MG, Orlandi A, Cervelli V. The effect of platelet rich plasma in hair regrowth: A randomized placebo-controlled trial. *Stem Cells Transl Med*. 2015 Nov;**4**:1317-23.
16. Dhurat R, Sukesh MS. Principles and methods of preparation of platelet-rich plasma: A review and author's perspective. *J Cutan Aesthet Surg.* 2014 Oct-Dec;**7**:189-97.
17. Aydin F, Pancar Yuksel E, Albayrak D. Platelet collection efficiencies of three different platelet-rich plasma preparation systems. *J Cosmet Laser Ther.* 2015 Jun;**17**:165-8.
18. Yin W, Xu H, Sheng J, Zhu Z, Jin D, Hsu P, et al. Optimization of pure platelet-rich plasma preparation: A comparative study of pure platelet-rich plasma obtained using different centrifugal conditions in a single-donor model. *Exp Ther Med.* 2017;**14**:2060-70.
19. Cervantes J, Perper M, Wong LL, Eber AE, Fricke ACV, Wikramanayake TC et al. Effectiveness of platelet-rich plasma for androgenetic alopecia: a review of the literature. *Skin Appendage Disord* 2018 Jan;**4**:1-11.
20. Dhillon RS, Schwarz EM, Maloney MD. Platelet-rich plasma therapy – future or trend? *Arthritis Res Ther.* 2012 Aug;**14**:219.
21. Garg S. Regeneration through platelet rich plasma – a cell therapy with a path full of milestones, controversies and cautions! *Indian Dermatol Online J*. 2021 Nov 25;**12**(Suppl. 1):S1-S3. doi: 10.4103/idoj.idoj_589_21. PMID: 34976875; PMCID: PMC8664168.
22. Arshdeep, Kumaran MS. Platelet-rich plasma in dermatology: boon or a bane? *Indian J Dermatol Venereol Leprol.* 2014;**80**:5-14.
23. Dohan Ehrenfest DM, Rasmusson L, Albrektsson T. Classification of platelet concentrates: from pure platelet-rich plasma (P-PRP) to leucocyte- and platelet-rich fibrin (L-PRF). *Trends Biotechnol.* 2009 Mar;**27**:158-67.

CHAPTER 4

THE ROLE OF PLATELET-RICH PLASMA IN VARIOUS TYPES OF ALOPECIA

CAROL LOBO, ANUVA BANSAL, SURUCHI GARG, AMI BADHEKA

Introduction

Hair loss is one of the most commonly presenting symptoms in dermatology outpatient departments in current times, resulting in considerable psychological disturbance and low self-esteem. Various treatment modalities have been tried in the management of alopecia. Despite the available therapeutic options, the search for new and more effective treatments is constant. PRP is a potentially useful therapeutic tool for alopecia, without major adverse effects.

History of PRP use in alopecia

PRP was first introduced in medicine as a haemostatic agent in surgery and for the management of chronic non-healing wounds[1,2] and was soon utilized in plastic surgery, orthopaedics and maxillofacial surgery due to its role in wound healing and tissue repair, and its anti-inflammatory properties.

Subsequently, PRP has gained importance in dermatology in the areas of scar revision, skin rejuvenation, wound healing and striae distensae.[3] Since 2006, PRP has been considered an effective therapeutic modality in alopecias for hair restoration.

The reasons for using PRP in alopecia

PRP consists of a plethora of growth factors and cytokines that stimulate the repair and regeneration of hair follicles.[4] These growth factors also facilitate angiogenesis and the development of adnexal structures.

Garg et al.[5] proposed a hair model termed "golden anchorage with 'molecular locking' of ectodermal and mesenchymal components, which is vital for the integrity and survival of hair follicle" (Figure 1). Golden anchorage comprises the ectodermal basement membrane, bulge stem cells and the bulge portion of the arrector pili muscle (APM). PRP works on this "golden anchorage" through its abundance of growth factors along with synergistic action on dermal papilla, keratinocytes, vasculature and neural cells, thus serving as an "elixir" for the hair growth.

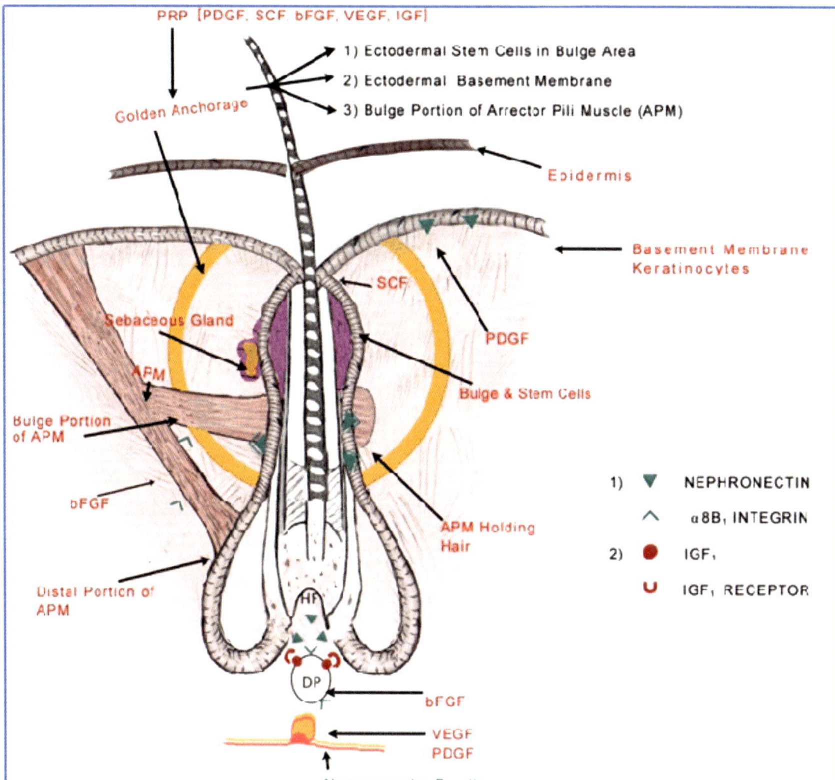

Figure 1: Golden anchorage model[5] Photo: Garg S, Manchanda S. Platelet-rich plasma – an 'elixir' for treatment of alopecia: personal experience on 117 patients with review of literature. *Stem Cell Investig.* 2017;**4**:64 (reproduced with permission)

Molecular signalling pathways/basis

PRP contains more than 20 growth factors that bind to stem cell receptors on hair follicle bulge stem cells.[6] The possible mechanisms by which PRP acts in androgenetic alopecia (AGA) may include any or all of a number of mechanisms as shown in Table 1.

Mechanism in alopecia areata

PRP suppresses the release of cytokines owing to its anti-inflammatory effects. It also increases the levels of Bcl-2 and Akt, both of which have anti-apoptotic effects.[8] The effect of β-catenin[11] and basic FGF[12] on melanin synthesis and the differentiation of melanocytes may explain the growth of pigmented hairs in alopecia areata through treatment with PRP.

Furthermore, it suppresses the release of MCP-1 (monocyte chemoattractant protein-1) and increases TGF-β expression, creating an anti-inflammatory environment around the hair follicle.[13-15]

Role in androgenetic alopecia

Androgenetic alopecia (AGA) is a hereditary androgen-dependent dermatological disorder which results in hair loss with a tendency to cause significant mental, social and psychological distress. It is characterized by the shortening of the anagen phase and progressive miniaturization of hair follicles. Despite the high demand for hair restoration, there are limited therapeutic options with varying efficacies. PRP has been explored as a treatment modality for AGA.

A review of literature by Cervantes et al.[16] evaluated the efficacy of PRP in the treatment of AGA in 12 studies and concluded that PRP increased terminal hair density and diameter, thereby promoting hair growth in most of the studies.

In a non-randomized study by Cervelli et al.[17] among 10 male patients all the outcome measures i.e. mean hairs, number of hair follicles, total hair density and epidermal thickness, showed statistically significant improvement at the end of three cycles of PRP. Additionally, an increase of Ki67+ was observed in the epidermal keratinocytes and hair follicular bulge cells.

A meta-analysis of seven studies among 194 patients by Giordano et al.[18] found a significantly increased number of hairs per square cm and thickness after PRP injections versus control.

Table 1: Molecular basis of PRP in AGA

Mechanism	Effector molecule/pathway
Prolongation of anagen phase	Insulin-like growth factor-1 (IGF-1)[7] Fibroblast growth factor-7 (FGF-7) Vascular endothelial growth factor (VEGF) Platelet-derived growth factor (PDGF) β-catenin
Development and differentiation of hair follicles	Wnt/β-catenin activation[8] Bcl-2[7]
Proliferation of hair follicle	FGF-7[7] Wnt/β-catenin activation[9] VEGF
Downregulation of hair follicle apoptosis	Extracellular signal-regulated kinase (ERK) and Akt signal pathway activation[8] Upregulation of Bcl-2[7]
Epidermal and hair follicle bulge cells proliferation	Ki-67
Angiogenesis and neovascularization in follicular area	VEGF [10] PDGF[7]

Most of the studies in the meta-analysis by Mao et al.[19] showed that subcutaneous injection of PRP was likely to increase hair diameter and density, and reduce hair loss in patients with AGA.

Zhou et al.[20] also concluded that PRP demonstrated excellent efficiency in the treatment of female pattern hair loss (FPHL) through hair density evaluation, in their extensive meta-analysis.

Histomorphometric evaluation in a study by Anitua et al.[21] showed significant improvement in epidermal thickness, perifollicular neoangiogenesis, terminal miniaturized hair ratio and decreased perivascular inflammatory infiltrates. Additionally, significant improvement was noted in hair diameter, mean hair density and terminal vellus hair ratio ($p<0.05$).

In an RCT[22] conducted among 26 patients with AGA, 13 patients were treated with PRP dalteparin and protamine microparticles (D/P MPs), and 13 patients with PRP and saline compared with the control (saline) were injected on the opposite side with equal hair density. Increased mean hair count and hair cross-section was noted in both PRP and saline and PRP and D/P MP treated areas compared to the areas treated with saline. Histological analysis of punch biopsy revealed increased epidermal thickness, the proliferation of fibroblasts and collagen fibres, and increased vasculature around hair follicles in both PRP, as well as PRP and D/P MP treated areas. No severe side effects were noted.

Sclafani[23] studied the effect of platelet-rich fibrin matrix (PRFM) on AGA in 15 subjects. After a series of three sessions of monthly intradermal PRFM injections, a significant increase in hair density indices was observed at 2 months ($p=0.0031$) and 3 months ($p=0.0277$) after the initial treatment.

In a study by Starace et al.[24] conducted among 10 patients with FPHL, increased hair density and diameter, and a decrease in vellus hairs were noted at 24 weeks compared to baseline with four sessions of fortnightly PRP.

Greco et al.[25] concluded in their study that PRP mesotherapy led to a significant increase in hair diameter and hair density among the five patients who received PRP therapy, compared to the five patients in the non-PRP group (a total of 10 patients with AGA).

Most of the studies found that PRP was a safe modality for the treatment of AGA with minimal side effects. The most common reported side effects were a mild headache and scalp tightness, which resolved without intervention within 24 hours.[26,27]

A few studies however noted slight to no improvement with PRP in AGA.[28-30] Mapar et al.[31] found no change in terminal hair count or vellus hair count in the PRP-treated group compared with the control group at 6 months. Another double-blind multicentre placebo-controlled study by Puig et al.[32] among 26 patients with FPHL, did not find any statistically significant difference between patients treated with PRP vs the placebo (normal saline) group.

Our experience

We studied the efficacy of three sessions of monthly PRP therapy in 65 male patients and 50 female patients.[5] Detailed video microscopic examination was conducted among 10 male and 10 female patients. New hair growth was noted at 4 weeks among male patients and by 6 weeks among females. An increase in hair count was noted in both groups. The increase in terminal hair count ($p=0.014$) and vellus hair count ($p=0.003$) was statistically significant among males. Additionally, improvement in hair density, perifollicular pigmentation, textural improvement of skin and multiplicity of hair in follicular units were noted.

Other significant studies on the use of PRP in the treatment of AGA are listed in Table 2.

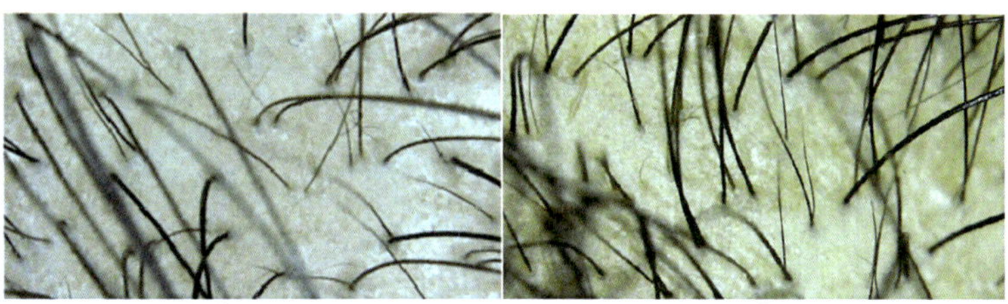

Before After

Figure 2: Male pattern hair loss with baseline image (total hair count of 40 hairs – 22 coarse, 15 intermediate and 3 vellus hairs, peripilar atrophic spots seen) and after (total hair count 55−47 coarse, 5 intermediate and 3 vellus hairs, no peripilar atrophic spots) three sessions of PRP therapy, 5% minoxidil and peptide solution, and nutritional supplements with increased early morning protein supply, yielding 30% increase in total hair count.

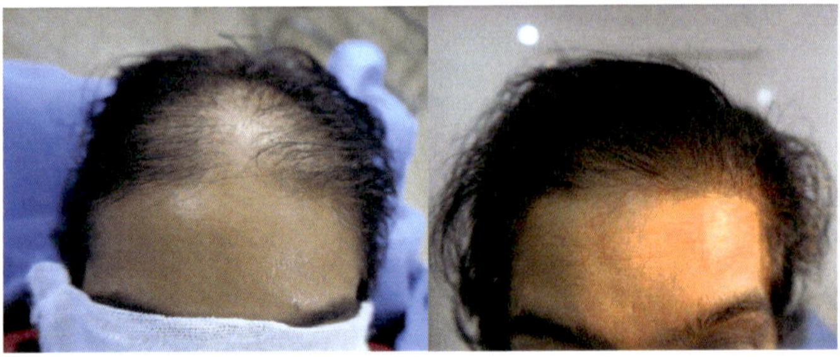

Figure 3: Female pattern hair loss treated with three sessions of PRP therapy, 2% minoxidil and peptide solution, and nutritional supplements with early morning increased protein supply and correction of vitamin D and B12 levels.

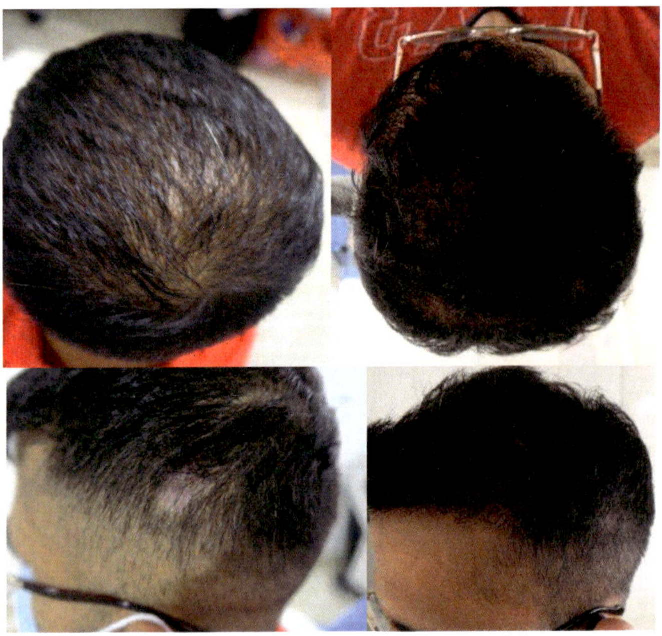

Before After

Figure 4: Male pattern hair loss with patches of the alopecia areata and diffuse thinning in parieto-occipital region and vertex treated with three sessions of PRP therapy, 5% minoxidil, tretinoin and azelaic acid solution along with nutritional supplements, early morning increased protein supply and correction of iron, vitamin D and B12 levels and counselling for reducing stress levels.

Table 2: PRP studies in the treatment of AGA

Study	Type of study	No of patients	Treatment	Treatment duration	Outcome
Verma et al.[33]	Prospective study	40 M*1 (30 completed)	Group A (n=16): PRP Group B (n=14): Minoxidil 5%	PRP: Once a month for 4 months Minoxidil: twice daily	Better outcome in Group A on global photography, hair growth questionnaire, hair pull test and patient satisfaction.
Hausauer[34]	Prospective, randomized, single-blind trial	40 (29 M*1 10 F*2 completed)	PRP	Group 1: once a month for 3 months and booster 3 months later Group 2: two sessions every 3 months	Significant improvement in hair count ($p<0.001$) and shaft calibre ($p<0.001$) at 6 months in both groups with a more rapid and profound improvement in Group 1 ($p<0.001$).
Alves and Grimalt[7]	Randomized placebo-controlled double-blind, half-head study	25 (11 M*1 11F*2 completed)	PRP vs saline Group A: 3 ml PRP on the right half of scalp and 3 ml saline on left half Group B: saline on both sides	Once a month for 3 months	Statistically significant improvements in mean telogen hairs, anagen hairs and hair density, in PRP-treated areas compared with baseline ($p<0.05$).

Gentile et al.[35]	Randomized placebo-controlled half-head group study	20 M*[1]	PRP on half scalp vs physiological solution as a control on opposite half	Once a month for 3 months	Statistically significant increase in mean hair count, total hair density ($p<0.0001$), and terminal hair density ($p=0.0003$) after 3 months with PRP compared to placebo. Increase in Ki67 + epidermal basal keratinocytes and hair follicular bulge cells in PRP-treated areas compared with baseline ($p<.05$).
Singhal et al.[36]	Prospective study	20: 8 M*[1], 2 F*[2] in each group	PRP vs medical treatment (control)	Once every 2 weeks for a total of four sessions	Clinical improvement in hair thickness, hair count, root strength and overall alopecia was seen in PRP group. The hair pull test showed a reduction by an average of 65%. No new hair growth or improvement in the hair pull test was noted among the controls.

Gupta et al.[37]	Open-labelled pilot	30 M*1	PRP	Once in 15 days for a total of six sessions	Increase in hair diameter and hair density was noted. Efficacy was higher in subjects with a shorter duration of disease and no family history of AGA.
Schiavone et al.[38]	Pilot study	64: 42 M*1, 22 F*2)	L-PRP* mixed with plasmatic proteins	Total of two sessions – baseline and 3 months later	Visible improvement in hair count and thickness after 6 months of PRP treatment. Approximately 40.6% of study participants attained a moderate level of improvement.
Gkini et al.[39]	Prospective cohort study	20: 18 M*1 2 F*2	PRP	Total of three sessions at intervals of 21 days Booster session at 6 months	Significantly increased hair density and thickness compared to baseline at 3, 6 and 12 months after PRP. ($p<0.001$). Norwood-Hamilton grade II–III responded better than more advanced cases.

Khatu et al.[40]	Prospective cohort study	11 M*1	PRP	Once every 2 weeks for a total of four sessions	Hair volume and coverage improved. Hair counts increased from 71FU** to 93FU**. The hair pull test was negative in nine patients after the fourth session.
Kachhawa et al.[41]	Placebo-controlled split head study	50 M*1 (44 completed)	PRP: left side of androgen-related areas vs saline: right side of androgen-related areas	Total of six sessions at intervals of 21 days	Increase in overall hair quality, thickness and density on digital image analysis and trichoscopy compared with baseline.
Tawfik and Osman[42]	Double-blind randomized placebo-controlled study	30 F*2	PRP vs saline in a selected area of scalp	Once a week for a total of four sessions; follow-up after 6 months	Statistically significant increase in hair thickness and density in PRP-treated areas compared with the control area and baseline at 6 months ($p<0.005$).
Butt et al.[43]	Prospective study	30: 20 M*1, 10 F*2	PRP	Total of two injections, 1 month apart	Increase in mean hair density, terminal vellus hair ratio and improvement in hair pull test at 6 months compared with baseline ($p<0.05$).

Kang et al.[44]	Prospective study	26: 15 M[*1] 11 F[*2]	13 patients (7 M[*1] 6 F[*2]): PRP 13 patients (8 M[*1] 5F[*2]): interfollicular placental extract control	Twice at three monthly intervals Placental extract: 1-week intervals for 6 months.	Clinical improvement in the mean number of hairs, and mean hair thickness was observed at 3 and 6 months post-PRP compared to baseline. A higher degree of improvement in treatment in hair thickness (p=0.027) and overall clinical improvements (p=0.023) was noted in the PRP group than in the group treated with the placental extract.
Sharma et al.[27]	Prospective case series	54: 49 M[*1] 5F[*2]	PRP with minoxidil (5% for males and 2% for females)	Total of three sessions at 6-weekly intervals	Improvement in hair density and the thickness of hair shaft, an increased number of hair follicles on dermoscopy. Reversal of response was noted in 12 (40%) patients. Improvement in female patients was comparatively less (24%).

Singh et al.[45]	Randomized double-blind placebo control trial	80 M[*1]	Group 1: Minoxidil 5% Group 2: PRP with minoxidil Group 3: Normal saline (NS) Group 4: PRP Placebo: 58 ml of NS and 2 ml spirit	PRP and placebo administered monthly for 3 months. Minoxidil: twice daily	Maximum improvement in hair density and patient satisfaction was noted in Group 2 followed by Group 4.
Shapiro et al.[46]	Randomized placebo-controlled split scalp	35: 18 M[*1] 17 F[*2]	PRP vs placebo	Once a month for 3 months	A significant increase in hair density in PRP-treated area vs saline compared to baseline at all visits was noted.
Rodrigues et al.[47]	Double-blind investigative pilot study	26 M[*1]	PRP vs control (saline)	Total of four sessions once every 15 days	Increase in hair density, hair count and percentage of anagen hairs was noted in the PRP group vs control and baseline.

Pakhomova et al.[48]	Comparative prospective study	69 M[*1]	Group 1: PRP Group 2: Minoxidil 5% Group 3: PRP + Minoxidil	Once a month for 4 months	PRP treatment was more effective than minoxidil monotherapy ($p=0.005$). Combination therapy was more effective than minoxidil monotherapy ($p<0.0001$) and PRP monotherapy ($p=0.007$). An increase in B-catenin and CD34 expression and a significant increase in Ki67+ index was noted following PRP injection.

*[1]M: Males * [2]F: Females * L-PRP: Leucocyte rich PRP **FU: Follicular unit

Role in alopecia areata

Alopecia areata (AA) is non-scarring alopecia characterized clinically by patchy areas of hair loss and histopathologically by peribulbar lymphocytic infiltrates responsible for pro-inflammatory cytokine release. Though intralesional steroids are the first line of therapy for adults with scalp involvement of less than 50%, they are notorious for local side effects like atrophy or telangiectasia. PRP in comparison is a safer modality of treatment in alopecia areata.

Singh et al.[49] noted relapse in only one patient among 20 patients of AA treated with PRP. There were no side effects, and the procedure was well tolerated.

Trink et al.[50] studied the effects of PRP in AA and found significantly increased hair regrowth and a decrease in the hair dystrophy, and burning and itching sensation in comparison to triamcinolone or the placebo. No side effects were noted during treatment.

In a study conducted by Balakrishnan et al.[51] a significant difference in severity of alopecia tool (SALT) score reduction after the second review was noted in the PRP group compared to the triamcinolone group ($p=0.028$). Excellent response was noted among 12.5% of patients in the PRP group after the final review, compared to none in the triamcinolone group.

Mubki[52] reported the positive synergistic effect of the combination of PRP with intralesional triamcinolone acetonide in a patient with long-standing AA.

Gupta et al.[53] reported successful management of a case of refractory alopecia totalis with PRP treatment in conjunction with intralesional triamcinolone and azathioprine. Similarly, Vekris et al. reported remarkable improvement of alopecia totalis with three sessions of PRP therapy in a case of twins with prior history of poor response to corticosteroids.[54]

PRP therapy has been useful in treating steroid-resistant forms of AA including ophiasis-type AA, and can be explored as a treatment modality in AA patients who develop side effects due to steroid injections.[55]

D'Ovidio and Roberto[56] evaluated the effect of PRP among 25 patients with severe chronic AA. Of the nine patients who completed the study, regrowth of terminal hair was noted among six patients and non-pigmented vellus hair was noted in the others at the end of the second session of PRP. Other studies of the use of PRP among AA have been listed in Table 3.

Table 3: PRP studies in alopecia areata

Study	Type of study	No of patients	Treatment	Treatment duration	Outcome
Singh et al.[49]	Prospective study	20	PRP	Once a month for 6 months	PRP was reported to be well tolerated. Relapse was reported in only one patient
Shumez et al.[57]	Non-randomized controlled study	74	Group 1 (n=26): PRP Group 2 (n=48): triamcinolone	Total of three sessions at three-weekly intervals	Remission was achieved in 53.8% of patients treated with PRP and 35.4% of patients with triamcinolone at the end of 6 weeks, though statistically not significant.
El Taieb et al.[58]	Randomized controlled study	90	Group A: minoxidil 5% solution Group B: PRP Group C: placebo	Once a month for 3 months	The PRP-treated group had significantly earlier hair regrowth, reduction in short vellus hair and dystrophic hair compared to minoxidil and control groups ($p<0.05$).

Role in telogen effluvium acute/chronic

There is a lack of literature on the efficacy of PRP in telogen effluvium. In our experience[5] a patient with telogen effluvium was managed with three sessions of once-a-month PRP and a significant increase in hair count and diameter was noted. An improvement in the skin texture and patient satisfaction score was also observed. Our personal experience with PRP therapy in post-COVID telogen effluvium (n=30), otherwise resistant to conventional therapy has been very rewarding. Nearly half (n=16) of the patients reported improvement in hair fall 7-10 days after the first session of PRP therapy. Ten patients reported increased fall for initial 2-3 weeks and subsequent improvement by the end of one month. Four patients continued to have ongoing hair fall though less severe than before. All the patients were offered oral micronutrient cyclical therapy, topical peptides, early morning plant-based protein supplements and correction of underlying micronutrients' deficiency was done based on blood tests.

Role in other alopecias

Petrov et al.[59] treated 20 cases of post-COVID anagen effluvium with three sessions of PRP and all patients had reduced hair loss after the second treatment and complete normalization after the third treatment.

Current Indian consensus guidelines

A 2019 expert consensus panel on the management of AGA in India[60] was of the view that patient selection for PRP is crucial and it should not be prescribed for all patients with AGA. Also, the panel concurred that the maximum duration of use of PRP is 6 months and long-term treatment is unsustainable. They recommended that PRP should be used as an adjuvant to minoxidil/finasteride rather than as a monotherapy.

The National IADVL PRP[61] task force has provided a clear consensus on the use of PRP in androgenetic alopecia. Use of the double-spin method at 100–300 g for 5–10 minutes followed by 400–700 g for 10–17 minutes using a microprocessor-controlled centrifuge with a brushless motor and swing-out rotor is ideal for the preparation of PRP. The ideal platelet concentration in PRP is 1 million to 1.5 million platelets/μl. Activation of PRP prior to injection into soft tissues is not required as the natural collagen type 1 acts as a natural activator. Additionally, glass vacutainers are preferred over plastic vacutainers for the preparation of PRP.

Pitfalls

The main disadvantages of PRP are pain during the procedure and slight scalp swelling and tightness post-procedure. Owing to its reversible effects, the major pitfall of PRP is the questionable sustainability over a period.

A few studies have shown a relatively poor response to PRP among patients with higher grades of AGA[37,39,62] and female AGA.[27,32]

Future advanced therapies

The next generation of autologous PRP is the inclusion of extracellular matrix (ECM) forming GF-ECM complex, which has been shown to demonstrate a synergistic effect in both human and equine wounds and holds a potential scope in hair restoration.[63]

Multipotent stem cells from the hair follicle and sebaceous glands are known to reverse the pathological mechanisms causing alopecia, and aid in the regeneration of complete hair follicles from the bulge stem cells.[64] Garg et al.[65] noted a remarkable improvement in the texture of hair, an increase in coarse terminal hair and a definite change in the hairline in a patient with androgenetic alopecia who was treated with five sessions of monthly PRP, followed by a single session of follicular stem cell suspension.

Conclusion

PRP has proved to be a safe and effective tool in the management of alopecia owing to its regenerative and regrowth potential. Further randomized controlled studies are needed especially in the lesser-explored areas of alopecia areata, anagen and telogen effluvium.

References

1. DelRossi AJ, Cernaianu AC, Vertrees RA, Wacker CJ, Fuller SJ, Cilley JH, et al. Platelet-rich plasma reduces postoperative blood loss after cardiopulmonary bypass. *J Thorac Cardiovasc Surg*. 1990 Aug;**100**: 281-6.
2. Cieslik-Bielecka A, Dohan Ehrenfest DM, Lubkowska A, Bielecki T. Microbicidal properties of leukocyte- and platelet-rich plasma/fibrin (L-PRP/L-PRF): new perspectives – *PubMed*. [no updated date; cited 20 November 2021] [Internet]. Available from:

https://pubmed.ncbi.nlm.nih.gov/23648198/
3. Arshdeep, Kumaran MS. Platelet-rich plasma in dermatology: Boon or a bane? *Indian J Dermatol Venereol Leprol* 2014;**80**:5-14.
4. Dhillon RS, Schwarz EM, Maloney MD. Platelet-rich plasma therapy – future or trend? *Arthritis Res Ther*. 2012 Aug 8;14:219.
5. Garg S, Manchanda S. Platelet-rich plasma – an 'Elixir' for treatment of alopecia: personal experience on 117 patients with review of literature. *Stem Cell Investig*. 2017 Jul 18;**4**:64-64.
6. Juhasz M, Sicco K, Shapiro J. The utility of platelet-rich plasma for the treatment of alopecia. *J Drugs Dermatol*. 2020 Jul 1;**19**:736-41.
7. Alves R, Grimalt R. Platelet-rich plasma and its use for cicatricial and non-cicatricial alopecias: a narrative review. *Dermatol Ther*. 2020 Aug;**10**:623-33.
8. Li ZJ, Choi H-I, Choi D-K, Sohn K-C, Im M, Seo Y-J, et al. Autologous platelet-rich plasma: a potential therapeutic tool for promoting hair growth. *Dermatol Surg Off Publ Am Soc Dermatol Surg Al*. 2012 Jul;**38**(7 Pt 1):1040-6.
9. Gupta AK, Carviel JA. Mechanistic model of platelet-rich plasma treatment for androgenetic alopecia. *Dermatol Surg Off Publ Am Soc Dermatol Surg Al*. 2016 Dec;**42**:1335-9.
10. Paus R. Do we need hair follicle stem cells and hair follicle neogenesis to cure common hair loss disorders? *Int Soc Hair Restor Surg*. 2008 May;**18**:81-90.
11. Luciani F, Champeval D, Herbette A, Denat L, Aylaj B, Martinozzi S, et al. Biological and mathematical modelling of melanocyte development. *Development.* 15 September 2011;**138**:3943–54. doi: https://doi.org/10.1242/dev.067447
12. Puri N, van der Weel MB, de Wit FS, Asghar SS, Das PK, Ramaiah A, et al. Basic fibroblast growth factor promotes melanin synthesis by melanocytes. *Arch Dermatol Res*. 1996 Sep;**288**:633-5.
13. Amable PR, Carias RBV, Teixeira MVT, da Cruz Pacheco I, Corrêa do Amaral RJF, Granjeiro JM, et al. Platelet-rich plasma preparation for regenerative medicine: optimization and quantification of cytokines and growth factors. *Stem Cell Res Ther*. 2013 Jun 7;**4**:67.
14. El-Sharkawy H, Kantarci A, Deady J, Hasturk H, Liu H, Alshahat M, et al. Platelet-rich plasma: growth factors and pro- and anti-inflammatory properties. *J Periodontol*. 2007 Apr;**78**:661-9.
15. Almohanna HM, Ahmed AA, Griggs JW, Tosti A. Platelet-rich plasma in the treatment of alopecia areata: a review. *J Investig Dermatol Symp Proc*. 2020 Nov;**20**:S45-9.

16. Cervantes J, Perper M, Wong LL, Eber AE, Villasante Fricke AC, Wikramanayake TC, et al. Effectiveness of platelet-rich plasma for androgenetic alopecia: a review of the literature. *Skin Appendage Disord*. 2018;**4**:1-11.
17. Cervelli V, Garcovich S, Bielli A, Cervelli G, Curcio BC, Scioli MG, et al. The effect of autologous activated platelet rich plasma (AA-PRP) injection on pattern hair loss: clinical and histomorphometric evaluation. *BioMed Res Int*. 2014;**2014**:1-9.
18. Giordano S, Romeo M, di Summa P, Salval A, Lankinen P. A meta-analysis on evidence of platelet-rich plasma for androgenetic alopecia. *Int J Trichology*. 2018;**10**:1.
19. Mao G, Zhang G, Fan W. Platelet-rich plasma for treating androgenic alopecia: a systematic review. *Aesthetic Plast Surg*. 2019 Oct;**43**:1326-36.
20. Zhou S, Qi F, Gong Y, Zhang C, Zhao S, Yang X, et al. Platelet-rich plasma in female androgenic alopecia: a comprehensive systematic review and meta-analysis. *Front Pharmacol*. 2021;**12**:726.
21. Anitua E, Aguirre JJ, Algorta J, Ayerdi E, Cabezas AI, Orive G, et al. Effectiveness of autologous preparation rich in growth factors for the treatment of chronic cutaneous ulcers. *J Biomed Mater Res B Appl Biomater*. 2008 Feb;**84B**:415-21.
22. Takikawa M, Nakamura S, Nakamura S, Ishirara M, Kishimoto S, Sasaki K, et al. Enhanced effect of platelet-rich plasma containing a new carrier on hair growth. *Dermatol Surg*. 2011 Dec;**37**:1721–9.
23. Sclafani A. Platelet-rich fibrin matrix (PRFM) for androgenetic alopecia. *Facial Plast Surg*. 2014 May 8;**30**:219-24.
24. Starace M, Alessandrini A, D'Acunto C, Melandri D, Bruni F, Patrizi A, et al. Platelet-rich plasma on female androgenetic alopecia: tested on 10 patients. *J Cosmet Dermatol*. 2019 Feb;**18**:59–64.
25. Greco J, Brandt R. The effects of autologous platelet rich plasma and various growth factors on non-transplanted miniaturized hair. *Hair Transpl Forum Int*. 2009 Mar 1;**19**:49-50.
26. Dubin DP, Lin MJ, Leight HM, Farberg AS, Torbeck RL, Burton WB, et al. The effect of platelet-rich plasma on female androgenetic alopecia: a randomized controlled trial. *J Am Acad Dermatol*. 2020 Nov;**83**:1294-7.
27. Sharma V, Bhari N, Patra S, Parihar A. Platelet-rich plasma therapy for androgenetic alopecia. *Indian J Dermatol*. 2019;**64**:417.
28. Marwah M, Godse K, Patil S, Nadkarni N. Is there sufficient research data to use platelet-rich plasma in dermatology? *Int J Trichology*. 2014 Jan 1;**6**:35.

29. Gressenberger P, Pregartner G, Gary T, Wolf P, Kopera D. Platelet-rich plasma for androgenetic alopecia treatment: a randomized placebo-controlled pilot study. *Acta Derm Venereol.* 2020;**100**: adv00247.
30. Borhan R, Gasnier C, Reygagne P. Autologous platelet rich plasma as a treatment of male androgenetic alopecia: study of 14 cases. *J Clin Exp Dermatol Res* 2015;**6**:292
31. Mapar MA, Shahriari S, Haghighizadeh MH. Efficacy of platelet-rich plasma in the treatment of androgenetic (male-patterned) alopecia: a pilot randomized controlled trial. *J Cosmet Laser Ther Off Publ Eur Soc Laser Dermatol.* 2016 Dec;**18**:452-5.
32. Puig CJ, Reese R, Peters M. Double-blind, placebo-controlled pilot study on the use of platelet-rich plasma in women with female androgenetic alopecia. *Dermatol Surg Off Publ Am Soc Dermatol Surg Al.* 2016 Nov;**42**:1243–7.
33. Verma K, Tegta GR, Verma G, Gupta M, Negi A, Sharma R. A study to compare the efficacy of platelet-rich plasma and minoxidil therapy for the treatment of androgenetic alopecia. *Int J Trichology.* 2019 Mar 1;**11**:68-79
34. Hausauer AK, Jones DH. Evaluating the efficacy of different platelet-rich plasma regimens for management of androgenetic alopecia: a single-center, blinded, randomized clinical trial. *Dermatol Surg Off Publ Am Soc Dermatol Surg Al.* 2018 Sep;**44**:1191-200.
35. Gentile P, Garcovich S, Bielli A, Scioli MG, Orlandi A, Cervelli V. The effect of platelet-rich plasma in hair regrowth: a randomized placebo-controlled trial. *Stem Cells Transl Med.* 2015 Nov;**4**:1317-23.
36. Singhal P, Agarwal S, Dhot P, Sayal S. Efficacy of platelet-rich plasma in treatment of androgenic alopecia. *Asian J Transfus Sci.* 2015;**9**:159.
37. Gupta S, Revathi TN, Sacchidanand S, Nataraj HV. A study of the efficacy of platelet-rich plasma in the treatment of androgenetic alopecia in males. *Indian J Dermatol Venereol Leprol.* 2017 May-Jun;**83**:412. doi: 10.4103/0378-6323.191128. PMID: 27679404.
38. Schiavone G, Raskovic D, Greco J, Abeni D. Platelet-rich plasma for androgenetic alopecia: a pilot study. *Dermatol Surg.* 2014 Sep;**40**:1010-9.
39. Gkini M-A, Kouskoukis A-E, Tripsianis G, Rigopoulos D, Kouskoukis K. Study of platelet-rich plasma injections in the treatment of androgenetic alopecia through a one-year period. *J Cutan Aesthetic Surg.* 2014 Dec;**7**:213–9.

40. Khatu S, More Y, Gokhale N, Chavhan D, Bendsure N. Platelet-rich plasma in androgenic alopecia: Myth or an effective tool. *J Cutan Aesthetic Surg.* 2014;**7**:107-10
41. Kachhawa D, Vats G, Sonare D, Rao P, Khuraiya S, Kataiya R. A spilt head study of efficacy of placebo versus platelet-rich plasma injections in the treatment of androgenic alopecia. *J Cutan Aesthetic Surg.* 2017 Jun;**10**:86-9.
42. Tawfik AA, Osman MAR. The effect of autologous activated platelet-rich plasma injection on female pattern hair loss: a randomized placebo-controlled study. *J Cosmet Dermatol.* 2018 Feb;**17**:47-53.
43. Butt G, Hussain I, Ahmed FJ, Choudhery MS. Efficacy of platelet-rich plasma in androgenetic alopecia patients. *J Cosmet Dermatol.* 2019 Aug;**18**:996-1001.
44. Kang J-S, Zheng Z, Choi MJ, Lee S-H, Kim D-Y, Cho SB. The effect of CD34+ cell-containing autologous platelet-rich plasma injection on pattern hair loss: a preliminary study. *J Eur Acad Dermatol Venereol.* 2014 Jan;**28**:72-9.
45. Singh S, Kumar V, Rai T. Comparison of efficacy of platelet-rich plasma therapy with or without topical 5% minoxidil in male-type baldness: a randomized, double-blind placebo control trial. *Indian J Dermatol Venereol Leprol.* 2020;**86**:150-7
46. Shapiro J, Ho A, Sukhdeo K, Yin L, Lo Sicco K. Evaluation of platelet-rich plasma as a treatment for androgenetic alopecia: A randomized controlled trial. *J Am Acad Dermatol.* 2020 Nov;**83**:1298-303.
47. Rodrigues BL, Montalvão SAL, Cancela RBB, Silva FAR, Urban A, Huber SC, et al. Treatment of male pattern alopecia with platelet-rich plasma: a double-blind controlled study with analysis of platelet number and growth factor levels. *J Am Acad Dermatol.* 2019 Mar;**80**:694-700.
48. Pakhomova EE, Smirnova IO. Comparative evaluation of the clinical efficacy of PRP-therapy, minoxidil, and their combination with immunohistochemical study of the dynamics of cell proliferation in the treatment of men with androgenetic alopecia. *Int J Mol Sci.* 2020 Sep 6;**21**:6516.
49. Singh S. Role of platelet-rich plasma in chronic alopecia areata: our centre experience. *Indian J Plast Surg.* 2015 Jan;**48**:057-9.
50. Trink A, Sorbellini E, Bezzola P, Rodella L, Rezzani R, Ramot Y, et al. A randomized, double-blind, placebo- and active-controlled, half-head study to evaluate the effects of platelet-rich plasma on alopecia areata. *Br J Dermatol.* 2013 Sep;**169**:690-4.

51. Balakrishnan A, Joy B, Thyvalappil A, Mathew P, Sreenivasan A, Sridharan R. A comparative study of therapeutic response to intralesional injections of platelet-rich plasma versus triamcinolone acetonide in alopecia areata. *Indian Dermatol Online J*. 2020 Sep 19;**11**:920-924. doi: 10.4103/idoj.IDOJ_6_20. PMID: 33344340; PMCID: PMC7734998.
52. Mubki T. Platelet-rich plasma combined with intralesional triamcinolone acetonide for the treatment of alopecia areata: A case report. *J Dermatol Dermatol Surg*. 2016 Jan 1;**20**:87–90.
53. Gupta S, Bisht PB, Kannan C. Alopecia totalis successfully treated with modified platelet-rich plasma therapy in a patient recalcitrant to traditional treatment modalities. *Clin Dermatol Rev* 2021;**5**:120-2.
54. Vekris A, Zafeiratou D, Andriopoulou A, Tsiatoura A. Total regrowth in chronic severe alopecia areata treated with platelet rich plasma: a case report and literature review. *Transpl Forum Int*. 2015;**25**:190-191.
55. Donovan J. Successful treatment of corticosteroid-resistant ophiasis-type alopecia areata (AA) with platelet-rich plasma (PRP). *JAAD Case Rep*. 2015 Sep;**1**:305-7.
56. d'Ovidio R, Roberto M. Limited effectiveness of platelet-rich-plasma treatment on chronic severe alopecia areata. *Hair Ther Transplant* 2014;**4** [no updated date; cited 20 Nov 2021] [Internet]. Available from: http://www.omicsgroup.org/journals/limited-effectiveness-of-plateletrichplasma-treatment-on-chronic-severe-alopecia-areata-2167-0951.1000116.php?aid=24661
57. Shumez H, Prasad P, Kaviarasan P, Deepika R. Intralesional platelet rich plasma vs intralesional triamcinolone in the treatment of alopecia areata: a comparative study. *Int J Med Res Health Sci*. 2015;**4**:118.
58. El Taieb MA, Ibrahim H, Nada EA, Seif Al-Din M. Platelets rich plasma versus minoxidil 5% in treatment of alopecia areata: a trichoscopic evaluation. *Dermatol Ther*. 2017 Jan;30. doi: 10.1111/dth.12437
59. Petrov A, Vasileva M. Effect of platelet-rich plasma on diffuse effluvium in post-COVID-19 infection. *Our Dermatol Online*. 2021;**12**:267-269
60. Mysore V, Parthasaradhi A, Kharkar R, Ghoshal A, Ganjoo A, Ravichandran G, et al. Expert consensus on the management of androgenetic alopecia in India. *Int J Trichology*. 2019;**11**:101-6.
61. Dashore S, Chouhan K, Nanda S, Sharma A. Preparation of platelet-rich plasma: national IADVL PRP taskforce recommendations. *Indian Dermatol Online J* 2021;**12**:S12-23.

62. Qu DS, Hu DZ, Zhang PY, Wang DP, Li DS, Huang DS, et al. Clinical studies on platelet-rich plasma (PRP) therapy for chronic cutaneous ulcers: a systematic review and meta-analysis of randomized controlled trials. https://home.liebertpub.com/wound. 2021 [no updated date; cited 25 February 2021] [Internet]. Available from: https://www.liebertpub.com/doi/abs/10.1089/wound.2020.1186
63. Clark RA. Synergistic signalling from extracellular matrix-growth factor complexes. *J Invest Dermatol*. 2008 Jun;**128**:1354-5. doi: 10.1038/jid.2008.75. PMID: 18478010.
64. Owczarczyk-Saczonek A, Krajewska-Włodarczyk M, Kruszewska A, Banasiak Ł, Placek W, Maksymowicz W, Wojtkiewicz J. Therapeutic potential of stem cells in follicle regeneration. *Stem Cells Int*. 2018; Aug 5;**2018**:1049641. doi: 10.1155/2018/1049641. PMID: 30154860; PMCID: PMC6098866.
65. Garg S, Saginatham H, Badheka A. Use of stem cells in intervention dermatology and trichology: a new hope. *J Stem Cell Res Dev Ther*. 2019;S1004.

CHAPTER 5

ROLE OF PLATELET-RICH PLASMA IN HAIR TRANSPLANTATION SURGERY

JILL CHITALIA, ANUVA BANSAL,
SURUCHI GARG

Hair transplantation surgery today is mainly practised as follicular unit extraction (FUE) more than follicular unit transection (FUT). The procedure involves harvesting hair follicles from the occipital area of the scalp and implantation into the frontotemporal or vertex area of the scalp in patterned hair loss patients. In burned-out cases of cicatricial alopecia, hair follicles are harvested from uninvolved areas of scalp and implanted into cicatrized patches of alopecia.[1]

The fate of hair follicle after transplantation

Once implanted into the scalp, hair undergoes an individual growth cycle. It first enters the catagen phase in the initial 2 weeks of implantation, which is characterized by an inflammatory process in which scalp redness and hair shaft shedding is common. The patient then enters the telogen phase for the next 3 to 4 months. This is followed by the latency period during which substantial follicular unit loss can occur because of apoptosis. Between 15% and 30% of the implanted grafts will be either eliminated or absorbed by the scalp. Therefore, only 70% to 85% of the implanted hair will finally enter the growing anagen phase.[2]

Factors affecting graft survival[3]

We can divide these factors into three main categories:

- follicle trauma
- vascular factors (oxygenation/revascularization)
- biochemical factors.

Follicle trauma happens during the surgery, when follicles can be subjected to transection, dehydration and crushing. The use of microscopes and follicular unit techniques minimizes transection.[3] Careful graft placement by less handling of the hair bulb and bulge area by an experienced surgeon will reduce crushing and damage to the graft. Keeping grafts moist throughout the process helps to prevent dehydration.[4]

Vascular factors include the successful revascularization of each graft. When this tissue is implanted back in the body it is re-exposed to oxygen, which triggers free radical production that may hamper graft survival ("ischaemia-reperfusion injury").[5]

Biochemical factors refer to the stress the hair follicles experience when they are kept out of the body for a period of time and then returned to the oxygenated graft bed. When tissue is outside the body, it undergoes "storage injury" due to the cut-off of oxygenated blood, lack of nutrients and temperature or pH shifts.[5]

Graft storage medium is an important factor of a hair transplant procedure

If the grafts are not stored properly, they may become dry or malnourished, and fail to grow when implanted into the scalp. Solutions with extracellular ionic balance such as normal saline, Ringer's lactate, tissue culture media and Plasma-Lyte A could make grafts in chilled storage more susceptible to electrolyte imbalance and cell swelling as sodium rushes into the cells. Intracellular type preservation solutions (Hypothermosol, Viaspan, Custodial) have a lower $Na+$ concentration, but are more expensive than extracellular balanced solutions. Many surgeons store grafts in normal saline, which mimics the normal chemistry (salt-to-water balance) of the blood plasma. While this storage medium may prevent desiccation, it lacks many of the nutrients the follicles normally receive from the scalp's natural blood supply.

To combat this problem and ensure grafts survival outside the body, some hair transplant surgeons are now using PRP or PRP-derived holding solutions.[2,6]

The role of PRP in changing the fate of hair follicles after HT

As PRP promotes cellular growth and healing, it has been investigated as an injectable hair loss solution. However, results with injectable PRP monotherapy were varied and somewhat controversial. Interestingly, researchers noticed that while PRP may not be a fully effective injectable hair loss treatment as a standalone therapy, it could still serve a twofold purpose in hair transplant surgery:[2,6,7] 1. PRP may serve as a viable storage solution for harvested follicular unit grafts before implantation and 2. injecting PRP into the recipient region after making the slits may promote faster healing and better growth.

The growth factors contained in the platelets of blood plasma are platelet-derived growth factor (PDGF), transforming growth factor (TGF), epidermal growth factor (EGF), fibroblast growth factor (FGF), insulin-like growth factor (IGF) and vascular endothelial growth factor (VEGF). They are protein molecules, which help in tissue angiogenesis and stimulate the healing and growth of new organic structures.[8-11]

The reasons for using PRP in outpatient surgical hair restoration are as follows:[12]

- to preserve and enhance hair follicle viability during and after hair transplantation;
- to induce early entry of hair follicles into the anagen phase;
- to promote and enhance tissue repair and healing after hair transplantation;
- to reinvigorate dormant hair follicles and stimulate new hair growth.

To preserve and enhance hair follicle viability

Donor hair follicle viability is preserved during the transition period by keeping the grafts in a storage solution that provides a protective environment of appropriate temperature, electrolyte balance and nutrient supply. Some surgeons recommend bathing of donor hair follicles in activated PRP just prior to transplantation.

Because PRP contains the body's natural blood plasma, growth factors and other molecules necessary for healthy follicles, it may lead to superior grafts and higher yield when used as a graft storage medium.[7]

Researchers have reported that PRP stimulates hair growth due to the action of platelet growth factors on hair follicle stem cells.[2] Stem cells are of ectodermal origin and produce epidermal cells and sebaceous glands. Germinative cells of the matrix, which are found at the dermal papilla, are of mesenchymal origin. These cells interact with each other and give rise to the future follicular unit, which consists of the hair shaft, sebaceous glands, arrector pili muscle and the perifollicular region. Authors have proposed a hair model termed "golden anchorage with 'molecular locking' of ectodermal and mesenchymal components for survival and integrity of hair follicle (HF)" in an already published article.[13] Golden anchorage comprises bulge stem cells, ectodermal basement membrane and the bulge portion of APM. PRP with its autologous supply of millions of growth factors works on golden anchorage along with keratinocytes (PDGF), dermal papilla (IGF and fibroblast growth factor), vasculature (VEGF and PDGF) and neural cells (nerve growth factor) in a multipronged manner serve as an "elixir" for hair growth.

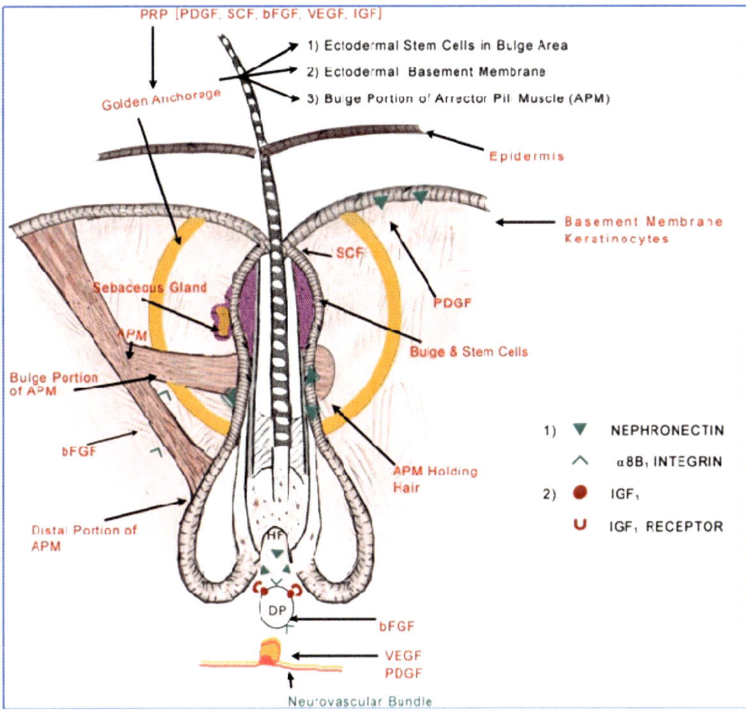

Figure 1: Golden anchorage model. Image: Garg S, Manchanda S. Platelet-rich plasma – an 'elixir' for treatment of alopecia: personal experience on 117 patients with review of literature. *Stem Cell Investig*. 2017;4:64 (reproduced with permission)

To induce early entry of hair follicle into the anagen phase

It is already known that hair growth depends on the induction of angiogenesis to fulfil the increased nutritional requirement of the rapid cell division of hair follicles during the anagen phase.[14] Vascular endothelial growth factor (VEGF) stimulates angiogenesis during development of the hair cycle. In 2001, Yano et al.[15] identified VEGF as a major mediator of hair follicle growth and cycling as it improves follicle vascularization, thus increasing the follicle size.

PRP increases anti-apoptotic Bcl-2 protein levels and prolongs survival of dermal papilla cells. Rinaldi et al.[7] reported this effect where they observed prolongation of the anagen and shortening of the catagen and telogen phases due to the effect of PRP released growth factors.

To promote and enhance tissue repair and healing

The receptor area of the scalp has perivascular inflammation and decreased capillary network that may hamper the survival and viability of the implanted grafts. Intradermal application of PRP could counteract this suboptimal environment as it has been reported to behave as an anti-inflammatory agent via the attenuation of the nuclear factor kB pathway by platelet releases growth factors.[16]

PDGF stimulates the migration of perivascular healing capable cells into a wound and controls the effects of other growth factors.[17] PDGF improves dermal regeneration, collagen synthesis and angiogenesis, and induces the expression of TGF-β.[18] TGF-beta plays a crucial role because it affects majority aspects of tissue wound repair, namely initiation and termination, and promotes differentiation and proliferation.[19]

In 2003, Carter et al.[20] reported that wounds treated with PRP gel exhibited enhanced wound repair and more organized collagen than control tissues, without excessive deposition of connective tissue or scar formation.

To reinvigorate dormant hair follicles

FGF and VEGF, present in high concentration in PRP, reduce fibrosis and induce neovascularization to normalize scalp milieu. Thus, PRP provides a conducive environment to stimulate activity in dormant hair follicles.[22]

Methods for using PRP during hair transplantation surgery[23]

For donor wound closure in FUT/ healing of donor area in FUE

After injecting PRP in the donor site, there is less bleeding and oozing post-operatively, faster healing and less scarring than those not treated with PRP.

In FUT, after the donor strip is harvested and the subcuticular layer is closed, activated PRP gel is injected into the wound from end to end, followed by the skin layer approximation with non-absorbable suture.

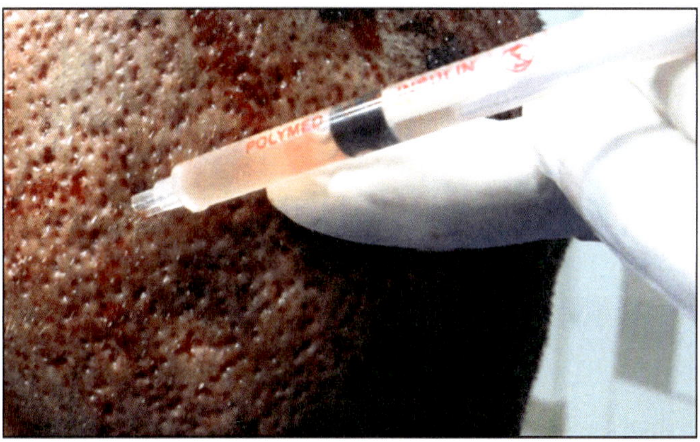

Figure 2: In FUE hair transplant, 0.05 ml of PPP is injected 1 cm apart in the occipital donor area from where the FUE grafts were harvested.

For storing harvested grafts

After the follicular units are harvested, they are bathed in an inactivated PRP solution (Figure 3). PRP may not require activation as collagen and thrombin act as spontaneous activators, though it can be activated with calcium chloride/thrombin or fibrinogen. However, it becomes a gel-like substance on activation and hair follicles become adherent to each other making them difficult to separate and be implanted.

Injection at recipient area

PRP is injected into the recipient scalp area after the graft pattern is completed to provide an enriched environment of concentrated growth factors, which help in faster healing of the wounds and promote angiogenesis for the newly implanted follicle growth. (Figure 4)

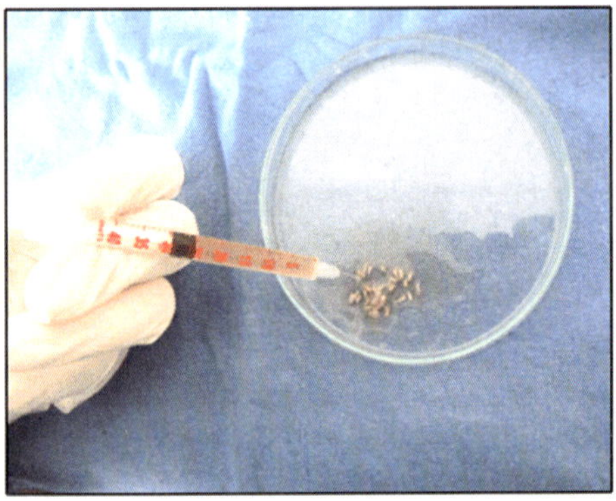

Figure 3: Bathing and storage of hair follicles in platelet-rich plasma

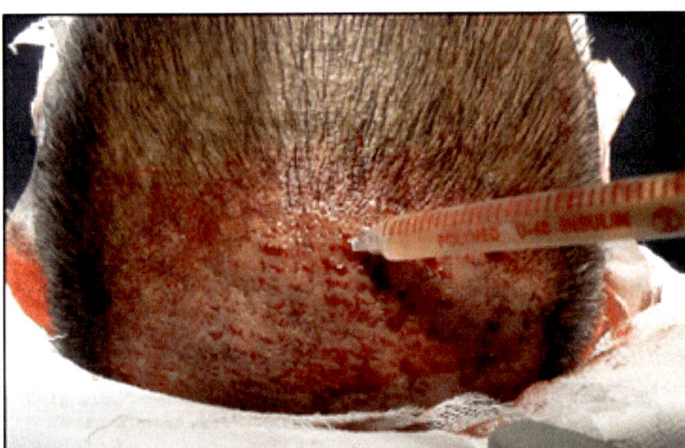

Figure 4: PRP injections during intraoperative period after creating slits (helps in activation of platelets and faster haemostasis) during FUE hair transplant

Efficacy of PRP combined with hair transplantation surgery (HTS)

Androgenic alopecia

There are only a few hair growth and survival studies using PRP in HTS. In the first study by Perez-Meza[6] in 2005, PRP was prepared with automated centrifuges and then used as a graft storage medium. The author recruited 10 patients in the study. Three boxes (1 cm^2 each) were marked on each side of the scalp for the PRP and placebo control, respectively. The grafts of the PRP group were preserved in the PRP solution (non-activated) and soaked in PRP gel (activated) 10 minutes before implantation. At the one-year follow-up, hair counts were similar between the two groups.

In 2006, Uebel[2] performed the second study using a manual centrifuge. He included 20 male AGA patients. Two areas of 2.5 cm^2 each were marked symmetrically on the scalp. Two groups of 180 follicular units were harvested and prepared – one group was stored with platelet plasma growth factors and the other was kept in saline solution. The follicular grafts were immersed in the platelet growth factor solution for 15 minutes to allow the growth factors to bind to the stem cells located in the bulge area. Then, 10 drops of 10% calcium chloride were added to the mixture for conversion of fibrinogen into fibrin, thereby producing the plasma gel that would seal the growth factors around the grafts. In both areas, grafts were implanted at 20 g/cm^2. After one year, the area treated with PRP demonstrated a yield of 18.7 FU/cm^2 vs. 16.4 FU/cm^2 of the placebo group, reporting an increase in follicular density of 15.1%. A recent randomized study with PRP and normal saline suggested an increase in density and hair growth stimulation when follicular units are pre-treated with platelet-rich plasma before implantation.[21]

Our experience

We published the study in 2016[22] in which 40 FUE hair transplant subjects were recruited in two groups (PRP and non-PRP) alternately. PRP was injected intradermally immediately after creating slits over the recipient area in the PRP group, and normal saline was used in the non-PRP group. Both groups were evaluated at 2, 4 and 8 weeks, and 3 and 6 months from the procedure.

In the PRP group, all subjects had >75% hair regrowth at 6 months, density of >75% of grafts was noticed in 12 patients at 4 weeks, indicating reduced fall of transplanted hair during the shock phase. New hair growth was visible at 8 weeks in 16 patients, and redness over the recipient area completely disappeared in 19 patients at 3 months from surgery. All subjects showed activity in dormant follicles as fine vellus hair besides the thick transplanted hair. (Figure 5)

In the non-PRP group, four patients had >75% hair regrowth at 6 months; none showed >75% graft density at 4 weeks, and 13 subjects showed dormant follicle activity at 4 months. The number of patients having longer hairs was significantly more in the PRP group. The study thus concludes that PRP therapy is beneficial in decreasing the catagen loss of transplanted hair and activating dormant follicles, thus increasing the rate of graft survival. It also helps in faster recovery of recipient area in FUE transplant subjects.

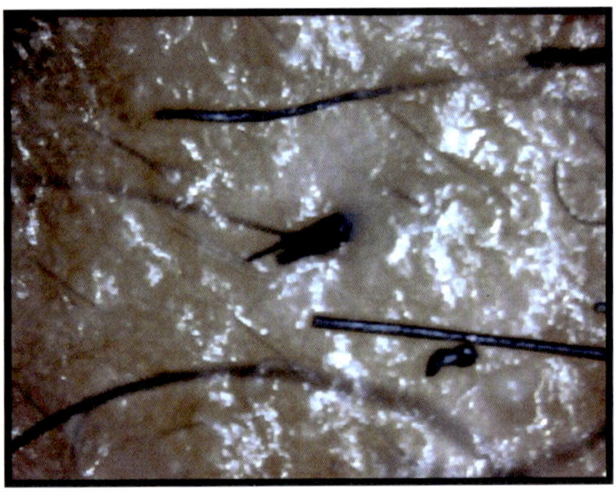

Figure 5: New hair follicle in the form of fine vellus hair after only 6 weeks in some cases post-transplant in PRP group

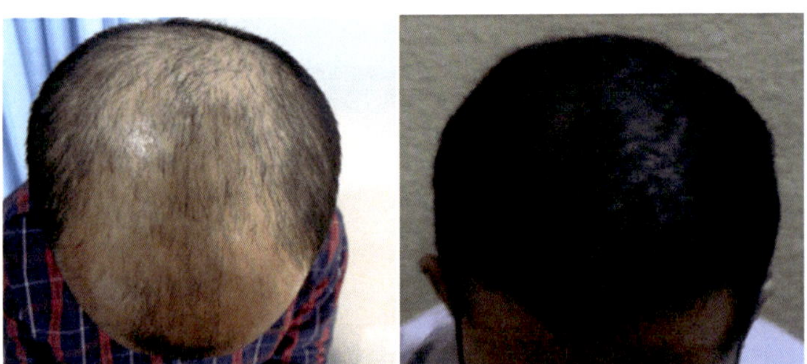

Figure 6: Pre and post 6 months' treatment results of Grade VI Hamilton-Norwood androgenetic alopecia treated with 4,500 FUE grafts along with injectable PRP therapy on two consecutive days, with oral multivitamin supplementation and 5% minoxidil solution without oral finasteride in the post-transplant period.

Injectable vs submersion technique

With injectable therapy in a study by Garg,[22] new anagen hair and activity of dormant follicles was observed at 2 months compared to 4 months in the study by Uebel et al.,[2] who used submersion technique. It may be deduced that spontaneous apoptosis of 15%–30% hairs can be reduced by injected PRP significantly.

The injected therapy could be better as there is earlier activity of dormant follicles and faster entry into the new anagen hair compared to the submersion technique.

Cicatricial alopecia

In 2016, Saxena reported a successful hair transplant outcome in cicatricial lichen planus of the scalp by combining scalp and beard hair along with platelet rich plasma.[24] PRP was injected intradermally into the recipient area just before graft implantation. A total of 900 hair follicular units equalling approximately 1,800 hairs at a density of 18 FU/cm^2 were transplanted, over two sessions. After transplant, topical 5% minoxidil application was advised. Ten months after the procedure, 80% of the transplanted grafts from both the scalp and the beard area survived and showed optimal growth, reasonably covering the alopecia patches. Compared to the scalp hair follicles, the transplanted follicles from the beard area showed faster hair growth.

Safety and complications of PRP

Since it is autologous, PRP is immunologically neutral and poses no danger of allergic, hypersensitivity or reactions to foreign bodies. A patient may experience a brief period of a burning sensation after application of a PRP gel. Inflammation may be associated with release of platelet-associated factors at the wound site or due to the effect of anticoagulant. The redness was more marked in our study in the initial 3 months and was explained on the basis of neovascularization, but it also aided faster healing in the PRP group.[22]

Conclusion

To summarize, PRP therapy improves the skin milieu of the recipient area to make it more receptive and fertile for newly transplanted hair by cell growth and differentiation, anti-apoptotic activity and neovascularization.

It also helps in providing a conducive environment for dormant hair follicles leading to their activity and appearance of new anagen hair as early as 2 months. PRP also helps in better healing and less scarring of the donor area.

Future prospects: ADSCs and dermal papilla cloning

In recent years, adult human hair follicle neogenesis has been an important subject in regenerative medicine. Up to the time of writing, two biological sources of follicular neogenesis have been researched:

1. Adipose-derived stem cells (ADSCs)
2. Human hair follicle stem cells

ADSCs

ADSCs have their own capacity of multidirectional differentiation, weak immunogenicity and lack of morbidity at the donor site. It has been reported that ADSCs secrete multiple growth factors – VEGF, FGFb, EGF, TGF and KGF (keratinocyte growth factor). Thus, they can enhance the wound healing process by promoting collagen synthesis and migration of dermal fibroblasts.[25] It is also shown that ADSC transplantation induces neovascularization to supply sufficient oxygen and nutrients to the newly formed tissue.[26] From these data, it would be rational to combine ADSC transplantation with PRP for better hair growth after hair transplantation surgery.

Human hair follicle stem cells

We know that dermal papilla cells play a crucial role in controlling the hair follicle growth cycle. It was demonstrated many years ago that adult rodent dermal papilla could be removed from the hair follicle and transplanted into recipient skin, where they were able to induce hair follicle neogenesis and hair growth.[27]

Currently we are conducting a randomized controlled trial of FUE hair transplant with injectable PRP versus follicular suspension with PRP therapy. Preliminary data suggest that the addition of follicular suspension, which is a source of stem cells, helps in the activation of secondary and tertiary hair roots in a native follicular graft which had otherwise miniaturized and were dormant and results are promising even at the 1-year interval, unlike PRP therapy where results start wearing off at approximately 1 year. (Figure 7)

Hair transplant procedures hold promising new prospects in light of tremendous work being done in regenerative medicine and trichology, and high-quality published literature is needed in this direction.

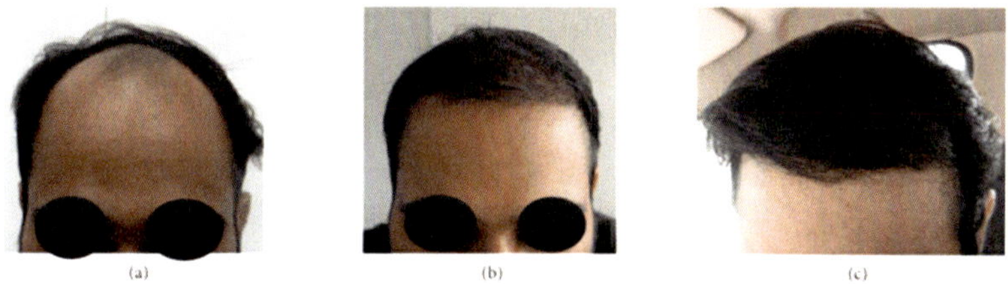

Figure 7: FUE hair transplant with PRP therapy and follicular suspension at baseline a) after 4 months b) and after a 1-year interval c). Noticeable filling effect at frontotemporal angles is seen at the 1-year interval though no oral finasteride was given after the transplant. Image: Garg S, Bansal A. Platelet rich plasma in intervention dermatology and trichology: How far have we come? Cosmoderma 2021;1:12[28]

References

1. Kutlubay Z, Kucuktas M, Engin B. Hair transplantation in the cicatricial alopecias. *Hair Ther Transplant*. 2013;**3**:109.
2. Uebel CO, da Silva JB, Cantarelli D, Martins P. The role of platelet plasma growth factors in male pattern baldness surgery. *Plast Reconstr Surg*. 2006;118:1458-66.
3. Parsley WM, Perez-Meza D. Review of factors affecting the growth and survival of follicular grafts. *J Cutan Aesthet Surg* 2010;**3**:69-75
4. Hwang SJ, Lee JJ, Oh BM, Kim DW, Kim JC, Kim MK. The effects of dehydration, preservation temperature and time on the hair grafts. *Ann Dermatol*. 2002;**14**:149-52.
5. Cooley J. Ischemia-reperfusion injury and graft storage solutions. *Hair Transpl Forum Int* 2004;**13**:121,127,130.
6. Perez-Meza D. Part II The use of autologous rich and poor plasma to enhance the wound healing and hair growth in hair restoration. In Programs and Abstracts. 13th ISHRS Annual Meeting 2005, Sydney, Australia
7. Rinaldi F, Sorbellini E, Coscera T. The role of platelet rich plasma to control anagen phase: Evaluation in vitro and in vivo hair transplant and hair treatment. *Int J Trichology*. 2011;**3**:514-5.
8. Converse JM, Uhlschmid CK, Ballantyne H. Plasmatic circulation in skin grafts: the phase of serum inhibition. *Plast Reconstr Surg*. 1969;

43:495.
9. Vogt PM, Lehnhardt M, Wagner D, Jansen V. Determination of endogenous growth factors in human wound fluid: temporal presence and profiles of secretion. *Plast Reconstr Surg*. 1998;102:117.
10. Bennett NT, Schultz GS. Growth factors and wound healing: biochemical properties of growth factors and their receptors. *Am J. Surg*.1993;**165**:728.
11. Steed, D. L. The role of growth factors in wound healing. *Surg. Clin. North Am*.1997;**77**:575.
12. Cooley J. Hair transplant graft survival and platelet rich plasma. http://www.regrowhair.com/hair-transplant-surgery/hair-transplant-graftsurvival-and-platelet-rich-plasma
13. Garg S, Manchanda S. Platelet-rich plasma – an 'elixir' for treatment of alopecia: personal experience on 117 patients with review of literature. *Stem Cell Investig*. 2017;**4**:64.
14. Rinaldi F, Sorbellini E, Bezzola P. Improving the revascularization of transplanted hair follicles through up-regulation of angiogenic growth factors. *Hair Transplant Forum Intl*. 2005;**17**:117-26.
15. Yano K, Brown L, Detmar M. Control of hair growth and follicle size by VEGF-mediated angiogenesis. *J Clin Invest*. 2001;**107**:409-17.
16. Anitua E, Pascual C, Perez-Gonzalez R, Orive G, Carro E. Intranasal PRGF-Endoret enhances neuronal survival and attenuates NF-jB-dependent inflammation process in a mouse model of Parkinson's disease. *J Controlled Release*. 2015;**203**:170-180.
17. Declair, V. The importance of growth factors in wound healing. *Ostomy Wound Manage*. 1999;**45**:64-68.
18. Ross, R. Platelet-derived growth factor. *Am Rev Med*.1986.38; 71-79.
19. Choi Y, Fuchs E. TGF-beta and retinoic acid regulation of growth and modifiers of differentiation human epidermal cells. *Cell Regul*.1990. 1; 791-809.
20. Carter CA, Jolly DG, Worden CE (snr), Hendren DG, Kane CJM. Platelet-rich plasma gel promotes differentiation and regeneration during equine wound healing. *Exp Mol Pathol*. 2003;74: 244-55.
21. Abdelkader R, Abdalbary S, Naguib I, Makarem K. Effect of platelet rich plasma versus saline solution as a preservation solution for hair transplantation. *Plast Reconstr Surg Glob Open*. 2020;**8**:e2875
22. Garg S. Outcome of intra-operative injected platelet-rich plasma therapy during follicular unit extraction hair transplant: a prospective randomised study in forty patients. *J Cutan Aesthet Surg*. 2016;**9**:157-64.
23. Greco J, Brandt R. Preliminary experience and extended applications

for the use of autologous platelet-rich plasma in hair transplantation surgery. *Hair Transplant Forum Intl*. 2007;**17**:131-132.
24. Saxena K, Saxena D Sawant S. Successful hair transplant outcome in cicatricial lichen planus of the scalp by combining scalp and beard hair along with platelet rich plasma. *Cutan Aesthet Surg.* 2016 Jan-Mar;**9**: 51-55.
25. Sheng L, Yang M, Liang Y, Li Q. Adipose tissue-derived stem cells (ADSCs) transplantation promotes regeneration of expanded skin using a tissue expansion model. *Wound Repair Regen*. 2013 Sep-Oct;**21**:746-54.
26. Lu F, Mizuno H, Uysal CA, Cai X, Ogawa R, Hyakusoku H. Improved viability of random pattern skin flaps through the use of adipose-derived stem cells. *Plast Reconstr Surg*. 2008 Jan;**121**:50-8.
27. Reynolds AJ, Jahoda CA. Cultured dermal papilla cells induce follicle formation and hair growth by transdifferentiation of an adult epidermis. Development. 1992 Jun;**115**:587-93.
28. Garg S, Bansal A. Platelet rich plasma in intervention dermatology and trichology: How far have we come? *Cosmoderma* 2021;**1**:12.

CHAPTER 6

PLATELET-RICH PLASMA IN CICATRICIAL ALOPECIA

ANKITA TUKNAYAT, ANUVA BANSAL, SURUCHI GARG

Introduction

Cicatricial or scarring alopecia is a generic term, which refers to patchy hair loss that occurs due to the permanent destruction of the hair follicles.[1] It may be primary when the disease process preferentially causes inflammatory damage to the hair follicles and spares the interfollicular reticular dermis, or secondary when the follicle is an innocent bystander and is damaged due to surrounding inflammation.[2]

There are many different classifications for primary cicatricial alopecia, either on the basis of the type of inflammatory cells or on the presence or absence of pustules.[2] The most common examples of scarring alopecia that we come across are chronic cutaneous discoid lupus erythematosus (DLE), lichen planopilaris (LPP), pseudopelade of Brocq and folliculitis decalvans. Treatment modalities are based primarily on the type of underlying disease process, and the progression of the disease. The various treatment modalities may be systemic or intralesional steroids, hydroxychloroquine, systemic retinoids, dapsone or thalidomide in diseases such as LPP and DLE, while systemic antibiotics and retinoids are the main line of treatment in diseases such as folliculitis decalvans and dissecting folliculitis of the scalp.[3] It is pertinent to note that the aim of all these treatment strategies is to stop the progression of the disease and none of these treatment modalities help in the regrowth of the hair that has been lost due to the disease. A multimodal treatment plan is required in most cases of scarring alopecia.

Platelet-rich plasma (PRP) is an autologous blood product that has been used in innumerable indications in orthopaedics, maxilla-facial and dental surgery, gynaecology, haematology, etc.[4-7] In dermatology, it has been used in pigmentary disorders, acne scars and facial rejuvenation, among other indications.[8-10] Its use has recently expanded to non-scarring alopecia such as androgenetic alopecia and alopecia areata.[11-14] Very few studies exist on the use of PRP in scarring alopecia.[15-18] It has been postulated to act through its multitude of growth factors to limit the disease process as well as to help in the regrowth of hair in scarring alopecia.

Pathogenesis of scarring alopecia

Hair follicles grow and recycle through the "bulge-activation hypothesis".[19] The stem cells of the follicle reside in the bulge region at the insertion of the arrector pili muscle (APM), which is the lowest permanent part of the follicle. At the end of telogen, these cells divide to give rise to transient amplifying cells that multiply to form the matrix cells. After this, the bulb disappears and the follicle enters telogen again to restart the cycle. The dermal papilla also has a pertinent role in that it moves upwards during telogen to interact with bulge cells to start their activation. These bulge stem cells are of ectodermal origin and express a number of extracellular matrix (ECM) proteins such as nephronectin, which acts as a link between epidermal cells and mesenchymal cells through its receptor a8β1 integrin.[20] Follicular stem cells are bipotent; they can form keratinocytes of the hair follicles as well as interfollicular epidermis.[21]

It is hypothesized that there are two types of follicles – primary follicles, which are in close intimate contact with APM – and secondary follicles, which are not in direct contact with the APM. APM plays a vital role in hair follicle morphogenesis and its renewal. It is said that it may be a source of stem cells to the follicle, thus secondary follicles are more susceptible to damage. It is believed that the deposition of nephronectin in the basement membrane creates a unique niche, leading to the attachment between the bulge region of the ectodermal hair follicle, mesenchymal APM and dermal papilla and this may prove to be a "golden anchorage" for hair follicle survival and integrity.[20]

Diseases such as LPP and DLE cause inflammatory damage to the bulge area of the hair follicle, thus leading to disruption in this golden anchorage and hair follicle cycling.[22,23] This leads to permanent destruction of the hair follicles, eventually leading to cicatricial alopecia.

Platelet-rich plasma

PRP is an autologous blood product that is rich in innumerable growth factors required for the homeostatic processes of the body. The active ingredient includes platelet alpha granules, which contain more than 30 growth factors such as platelet-derived growth factor (PDGF), transforming growth factor-β (TGF-b), epidermal growth factor (EGF), fibroblast growth factor (FGF) and vascular endothelial growth factor (VEGF).[16] These growth factors stimulate cells such as osteoblasts, adult mesenchymal stem cells, endothelial cells, fibroblasts and epidermal cells, thus promoting tissue healing, angiogenesis, collagen synthesis, matrix formation and osteoid production.[24]

Mechanism of action of PRP in cicatricial alopecia

PRP acts at various steps of the pathogenesis of scarring alopecia. It has four predominant actions:

Anti-inflammatory

This is the most important action of PRP that targets the underlying pathophysiology of scarring alopecia. Growth factors such as VEGF and hepatocyte growth factor (HGF) contained in platelet granules target various signal transduction pathways leading to a decrease in inflammation.[25] PRP also decreases NF-kB signalling, which further reduces COX-1, COX-2 and prostaglandins leading to decreased inflammation. In addition to these, PRP also contains IL-1 receptor antagonists IL-4, IL-10 and TGF-b, which further leads to its anti-phlogistic activity. It also inhibits macrophage chemotactic factor 1 (MCP-1).[24]

Regenerative properties

It contains many growth factors such as insulin-like growth factor (IGF-1) and basic fibroblast growth factor (bFGF), which activate protein kinase B and the extracellular signal-regulated kinase (ERK) pathway, which leads to decreased degradation of beta-catenin. Beta-catenin helps in preserving follicular stem cells and thus promotes hair follicle growth.[25-27]

Anti-apoptotic

This effect is predominantly due to the activating effect of FGF on the beta-catenin pathway and versican, which leads to improved survival of hair follicles. Another reason for the anti-apoptotic effect of PRP is due to its inhibition of Bcl-2 associated death receptor pathway. VEGF acts as an anti-apoptotic as well as a pro-angiogenetic factor.[27]

Antimicrobial effect

Platelets participate in antibody-dependent cell cytotoxicity functions to kill pathogens. Platelet granules release platelet-activating factor, C5 protease, platelet factor-4 and free radicals, which have an antimicrobial role. Platelets granules also secrete PMPs (platelet microbicidal protein), tPMPs (thrombin-induced PMPs), and B-lysin, which have a direct microbicidal effect. These PMPs also potentiate the antimicrobial effect of antibiotics.

PRP also decreases pruritus and thus improves the quality of life in patients.[28-31] PRP exhibits molecular locking of ectodermal and mesenchymal components for the survival and integrity of hair follicles.[20] It boosts keratinocytes, dermal papilla cells and nerve cells. It also promotes angiogenesis and to add to all these effects, it also acts as an anti-inflammatory agent. All these properties make it a multipurpose potion for the nutrition and growth of hair follicles (Figure 1).

PRP has regenerative properties as well as antimicrobial, anti-inflammatory and anti-apoptotic effects. Early initiation of combination treatment of PRP along with immunomodulators may serve a role in a remarkable response in patients with cicatricial alopecia.

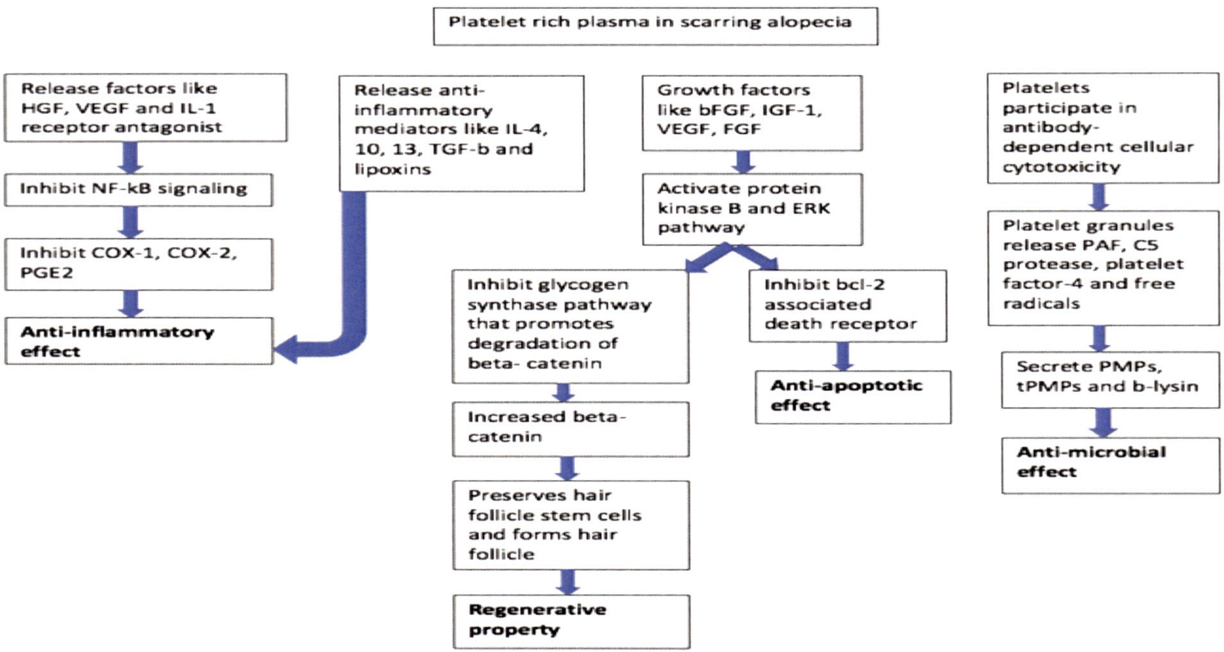

Figure 1: Role of PRP in scarring alopecia

Previous studies

Dina et al. used PRP in two patients with primary cicatricial alopecia and observed an improvement in hair density in both cases.[15] Suh et al. used PRP in two patients with folliculitis decalvans who showed successful symptom control after three sessions.[16] Özcan et al. successfully used PRP in a patient with frontal fibrosing alopecia and reported improvement of perifollicular erythema, scaling and lichenoid papules on the frontotemporal hairline in a case with frontal fibrosing alopecia with five sessions of PRP injected into the frontotemporal hairline and eyebrows of the patient.[17] In a study by Fakahany et al., one case each of cicatricial alopecia and traction alopecia were treated with 20 sessions of automated microneedling combined with PRP, every two weeks.[18] Marked clinical improvement with variable degrees of patient satisfaction was reported. Though all these studies have a few patients, the results are promising.

Methods of preparing PRP

A number of protocols are available for the production of PRP. All of these involve a centrifugation process which may be manual or automated. The volume of the blood sample taken, the anticoagulants used, the number of centrifugations, and the respective time and centrifugal force differ in different protocols. The most commonly used method has been described below.

Ten millilitres of venous blood is withdrawn by means of a wide bore needle and a vacutainer containing an anticoagulant. Commonly used anticoagulants include heparin, citrate, acid citrate dextrose (ACD), and citrate theophylline adenosine dipyridamole (CTAD). Double centrifugation method is used. The first centrifugation is slow to avoid gyrating down platelets and to isolate plasma, and is run for 10 minutes at 1,600 rpm. The supernatant plasma along with the buffy coat is withdrawn and re-centrifuged. A second centrifugation is done for 10 minutes at 4,000 rpm, after which the platelets separate and form a greyish pellet at the bottom of the tube, the rest being platelet-poor plasma. About 1 ml of this platelet-poor plasma is decanted off and the platelet pellet is re-suspended in the remaining plasma to produce PRP. With 10 ml of blood, about 1–1.5 ml of PRP is obtained.[4]

The optimum concentration of platelets in PRP has been found to be 2.5 times the baseline. Though there is lot of controversy but above this concentration, there are no added advantages – rather, it may be disadvantageous.[4] PRP activation prior to injection is another parameter that requires further discussion. Activation of platelets in PRP results in rapid growth factor release, with 90% of the prefabricated factors released in 10 minutes. Many growth factors have short half-lives, so the greatest efficacy may result if they are activated at or just prior to injection. PRP can be activated exogenously by mechanical trauma, thrombin or calcium chloride. Once PRP is activated, a fibrin network begins to form, solidifying the plasma and creating a fibrin clot or membrane. If PRP is activated too strongly, the fibrin network will be an unstable, bivalent network. A tetramolecular stable network forms if it is activated in a more physiologic manner.[9] Although this can be useful for surgical procedures, it is undesirable to have the PRP overly viscous when injecting into soft tissue or skin. Thus, most protocols use large-bore needles (>22) to draw the blood and re-inject PRP to avoid unintentional activation of platelets.[5]

Authors use Renew cell kits or Ycell bio kits and single-spin method for 10ml blood mixed with 1.5 ml ACD-A, centrifuged at 3400 rpm, 1350 RCF for 4 minutes. This method gives 3−4 times concentration of platelets from the baseline.

Some centrifuges offer specific braking mechanisms to prevent unintentional activation. The optimal regimen to prevent unintentional activation is not clear. PRP, when used in soft tissue, does not need to be exogenously activated as collagen is a natural activator of PRP. Heat also activates PRP so the preparation room temperature should be around 20–22 degrees to avoid unintentional activation of PRP; temperature-controlled centrifuges can be used for better efficacy.[8] If prepared using a sterile technique, platelets remain viable and sterile for up to 8 hours.

Modes of delivery of PRP in alopecia

As a standalone treatment, PRP can be injected intradermally by the nappage technique, or it may be used with microneedling. In patients with scarring where all treatments have failed, a hair transplant can be tried. Hair transplant as a standalone treatment leads to lower success rates as the graft uptake is poor, due to fibrosis and decreased vascularity in the recipient area. PRP-induced production of angiogenic GFs helps improve the cutaneous ischaemic conditions via perifollicular neovascularization. In a study by Saxena et al., 1 ml of PRP injected intradermally into the recipient area prior to graft implantation resulted in a successful hair transplant outcome in the cicatricial lichen planus of the scalp. PRP with its potential to improve the vascularity and regenerate the scarred tissue, making it more receptive, can serve as an adjuvant to hair transplant in compromised recipient areas as seen in scarring alopecia.[32]

Thus, PRP can be used along with hair transplants in such patients to improve graft uptake.

Adverse effects

Being autologous, the adverse effects of PRP therapy are rare and minimal, and include pain in the injected area, infection, skin discoloration, allergic reaction and blood clot formation.[33] There have been very few case reports of severe allergic reactions to PRP.[34-37] It is hypothesized that it may be due to calcium chloride or thrombin used to activate it before use. Some patients may develop transient regional lymphadenopathy due to exaggerated immune response induced by leukocytes and monocytes present in PRP.[36]

Contraindications

Absolute contraindications[10]:

- platelet dysfunction syndrome and critical thrombocytopenia;*
- haemodynamic instability;
- septicaemia;**
- local infection at the site of the procedure;
- patient unwilling to accept risks.

Relative contraindications[33]

- consistent use of non-steroidal anti-inflammatory drugs (NSAIDs) within 48 hours of the procedure;
- corticosteroid injection at a treatment site within one month;
- systemic use of corticosteroids within two weeks, causing a pro-coagulant state which may result in an aberrant response to PRP;
- tobacco use;
- recent fever or illness;
- cancer – especially of haematopoietic or bone tissue;***
- HGB < 10 g/dl;
- platelet count $< 10^5$/ul.

* Anticoagulants used to prepare PRP such as citrate, theophylline, adenosine and CTAD are specific inhibitors of platelet function. Theophylline and dipyridamole

inhibit cAMP phosphodiesterase activity and adenosine stimulates membrane adenylyl cyclase, which consequently leads to an increase in platelet cAMP and inhibition of calcium-mediated responses leading to a reduction in platelet activation. Thus, PRP is contraindicated in patients who already have low or dysfunctional platelets.[35]
** As PRP enhances chemotaxis, in patients with septic shock who are already in a condition of cytokine storm, it may lead to sudden deterioration.
***There is a controversial risk of growth factors in PRP inducing cellular proliferation and thus increasing cancer risk, but this seems more of a theoretical risk.

Our experience

Garg et al. used PRP along with follicular unit extraction (FUE) in patients with lichen sclerosus et atrophicus (LSEA) and showed a good graft survival four months after treatment.[20]

The author performed a combination of punch grafting with 2 mm diameter biopsy punches to transplant around 25 grafts with intraoperative PRP therapy in a patient with stable LSEA of four-year duration. Post-procedure evaluation at four months revealed that all the grafts were surviving well. Thus, in our opinion, in cases of cicatricial alopecia scarcity of ostia might be associated with reduced chances of the reversal of damaged hair follicles, and the transplant of new follicles through punch grafting can serve as a vital source of stem cells, arrector pili muscle, epidermal basement membrane as well as nerve bundle. Subsequent FUE hair transplant will be well taken up due to normal skin texture and will help in restoring the hair density and improve the cosmetic outcome.

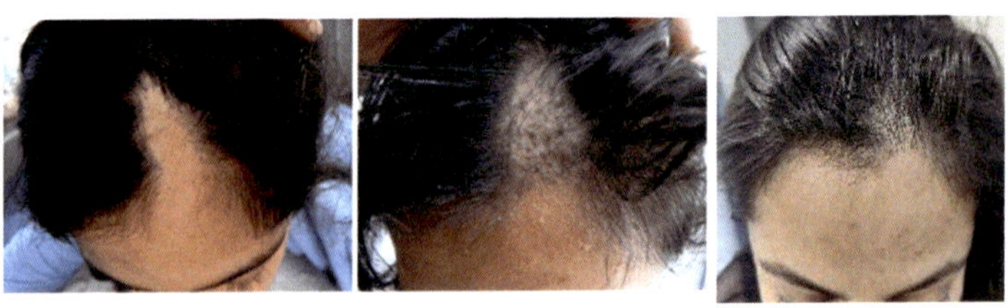

Figure 2: Pre- and post-procedural photographs (at baseline, at 4 months and after 7 years) of a patient with stable lichen sclerosus et atrophicus (LSEA) of four years' duration who was managed with punch grafting with intraoperative injectable PRP. The density can be further improved with subsequent sessions of FUE hair transplant with injectable PRP therapy.
Photo: Garg & Manchanda.[20]

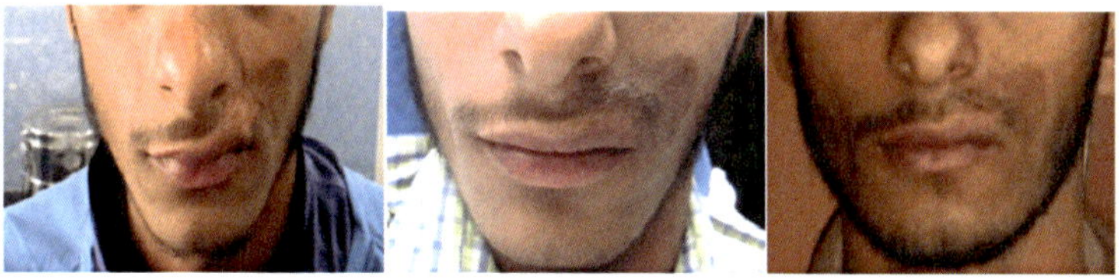

Figure 3: Post-burn scarring alopecia over moustache, baseline, after four months and after seven years treated with FUE hair transplant and PRP injections along with Er:YAG resurfacing. Photo: Garg et al[37].[38]

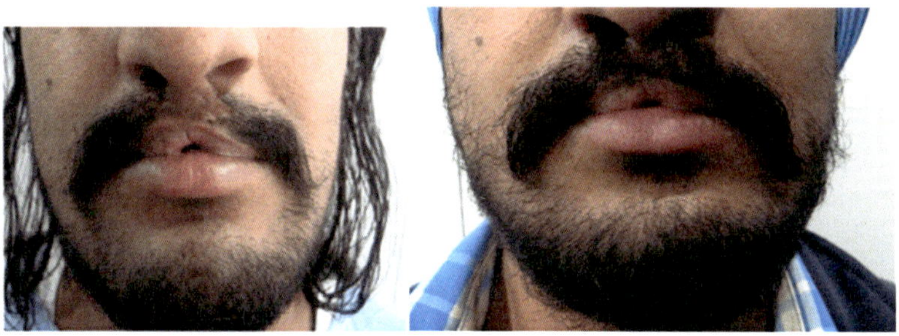

Figure 4: Post cleft lip surgery scar after four months of treatment with FUE hair transplant and PRP injections over scar and in the upper lip. Photo: Garg et al.[38]

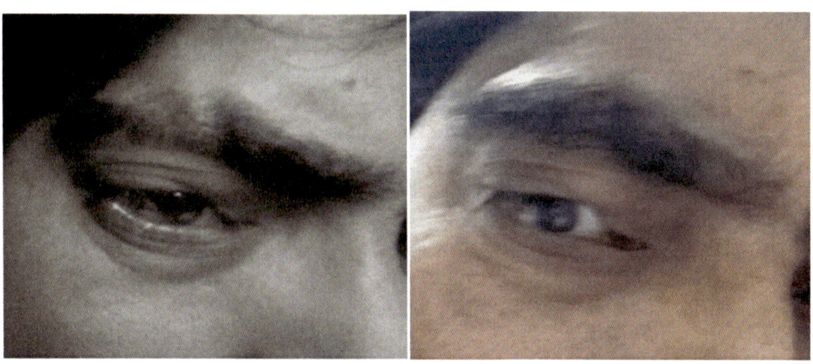

Figure 5: Post-traumatic scar over eyebrow treated with FUE hair transplant and PRP injections after five months of treatment.[38] Photo: Garg et al.[38]

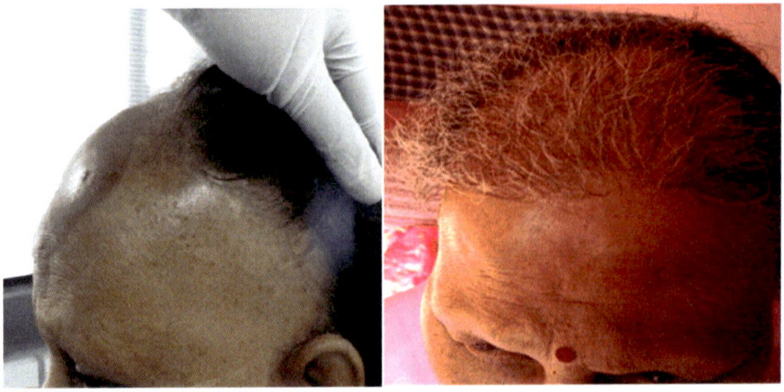

Figure 6: Frontal fibrosing alopecia treated with FUE hair transplant and PRP injections after eight months of surgery. Photo: Garg et al.[38]

Conclusion

PRP has a definite role in scarring alopecia due to its anti-inflammatory, regenerative, anti-apoptotic and antimicrobial properties. The various anti-inflammatory, pro-angiogenic cytokines present in PRP may help diminish the inflammation, protecting and stimulating the new follicle in cicatricial alopecia. There is a high probability that introduction of these growth factors results in ongoing repair and normalizes the environment of treated area over subsequent years, as was shown in documented cases. Early initiation of combination treatment of PRP along with immuno-modulators may serve a role in a remarkable response in patients with cicatricial alopecia.

References

1. Ross EK, Tan E, Shapiro J. Update on primary cicatricial alopecias. *J Am Acad Dermatol.* 2005;**53**:1-37.
2. Tan E, Martinka M, Ball N, Shapiro, J. Primary cicatricial alopecias: clinicopathology of 112 cases. *J Am Acad of Dermatol*. 2004;**50**:25-32. 10.1016/j.jaad.2003.04.001.
3. Somani N, Bergfeld WF. Cicatricial alopecia: classification and histopathology. *Dermatol Ther*. 2008;**21**:221-37.
4. International Cellular Medicine Society Guidelines for PRP: Section VIII: platelet rich plasma (PRP) guidelines. Las Vegas (NV): International Cellular Medicine Society; 2011. [No updated date; cited 29 May 2020] [Internet]. Available from:

http://www.cellmedicinesociety.org/attachments/370_Section%2010%20-%20Platelet%20Rich%20Plasma%20(PRP)%20Guidelines.pdf.
5. Anitua E, Prado R, Sánchez M, Orive G. Platelet-rich plasma: preparation and formulation. *Oper Tech Orthop.* 2012; **22**:25-32.
6. Eppley BL, Pietzak WS, Blanton M. Platelet-rich plasma: a review of biology and applications in plastic surgery. *Plast Reconstr Surg*. 2006; **118**:147-159.
7. Marx RE. Platelet-rich plasma: evidence to support its use. *J Oral Maxillofac Surg.* 2004;**62**:489-96.
8. Tuknayat A, Thami GP, Bhalla M, Sandhu JK. Autologous intralesional platelet rich plasma improves melasma. *Dermatol Ther*. 2021 Mar;**34**:e14881.
9. Lynch MD, Bashir S. Applications of platelet-rich plasma in dermatology: a critical appraisal of the literature. *J Dermatolog Treat*. 2016;**27**:285-9.
10. Tuknayat A, Bhalla M, Thami GP. Platelet-rich plasma is a promising therapy for melasma. *J Cosmet Dermatol.* 2021;**20**: 2431-6.
11. Picard F, Hersant B, Niddam J, Meningaud J-P. Injections of platelet-rich plasma for androgenic alopecia: a systematic review. *J Stomatol Oral Maxillofac Surg.* 2017;**118**:291-7.
12. Anitua E, Pino A, Martinez N, Orive G, Berridi D. The effect of plasma rich in growth factors on pattern hair loss: a pilot study. *Dermatol Surg* 2017;**43**:658-70.
13. Li ZJ, Choi HI, Choi DK, Sohn KC, Im M, Seo YJ, et al. Autologous platelet-rich plasma: a potential therapeutic tool for promoting hair growth. *Dermatol Surg.* 2012;**38**:1040-6.
14. Trink A, Sorbellini E, Bezzola P, Rodella L, Rezzani R, Ramoy Y, et al. A randomized, double-blind, placebo- and active-controlled, half-head study to evaluate the effects of platelet-rich plasma on alopecia areata. *Br J Dermatol.* 2013;**169**:690-4. 10.1111/bjd.12397
15. Dina Y, Aguh C. Use of platelet-rich plasma in cicatricial alopecia. *Dermatol Surg.* 2019;**45**:979-81.
16. Suh S, Nguyen C, Zhao L, Mesinkovska NA. The role of platelet-rich plasma therapy in refractory folliculitis decalvans. *JAAD Case Rep.* 2021;**12**:85-87. doi:10.1016/j.jdcr.2021.04.008
17. Özcan D, Vural AT, Özen Ö. Platelet-rich plasma for treatment resistant frontal fibrosing alopecia: a case report. *Dermatol Ther*. 2019;**23**:e 13072.
18. Fakahany H, Raouf H, Medhat W. Using automated microneedling with platelet rich plasma for treating cicatricial alopecia, recalcitrant

alopecia areata and traction alopecia, case report. *J Am Acad Dermatol* 2016;**74**;5:140.
19. Sun TT, Cotsarelis G, Lavker RM. Hair follicular stem cells: the bulge-activation hypothesis. *J Invest Dermatol.* 1991;**96**:77S-78S. doi: 10.1111/1523-1747.ep12471959.
20. Garg S, Manchanda S. Platelet-rich plasma – an 'elixir' for treatment of alopecia: personal experience on 117 patients with review of literature. *Stem Cell Investig.* 2017;**4**:64.
21. Bhang SH, Cho S-W, Lim JM, Kang JM, Lee T-J, Yang HS, et al. Locally delivered growth factor enhances the angiogenic efficacy of adipose-derived stromal cells transplanted to ischemic limbs. *Stem Cells.* 2009;**27**:1976-86.
22. Bolanča Ž, Goren A, Getaldić-Švarc B, Vučić M, Šitum M. Platelet-rich plasma as a novel treatment for lichen planopillaris. *Dermatol Ther.* 2016;**29**:233-5.
23. Jha AK. Platelet-rich plasma as an adjunctive treatment in lichen planopilaris. *J Am Acad Dermatol.* 2019;**80**:e109-e110.
24. El-Sharkawy H, Kantarci A, Deady J, Hasturk H, Liu H, Alshahat M, et al. Platelet-rich plasma: growth factors and pro- and anti-inflammatory properties. *J Periodontol.* 2007;**78**:661-9.
25. Zhang J, Middleton KK, Fu FH, Im H-J, Wang JH-C. HGF mediates the anti-inflammatory effects of PRP on injured tendons. *PLoS ONE* 2013;**8**:e67303. doi:10.1371/journal.pone.0067303.
26. Bendinelli P, Matteucci E, Dogliotti G, Corsi Romanelli M, Banfi G, Maroni P, et al. Molecular basis of anti-inflammatory action of platelet-rich plasma on human chondrocytes: mechanisms of NF-kappa B inhibition via HGF. *J Cell Physiol.* 2010;**225**:757-66.
27. Anitua E, Andia I, Ardanza B, Nurden P, Nurden AT. Autologous platelets as a source of proteins for healing and tissue regeneration. *Thromb Haemost* 2004;**91**:4-15.
28. Yeaman MR. The role of platelets in antimicrobial host defense. *Clin Infect Dis.* 1997;**25**:951-968 [quiz: 969-970].
29. Drago L, Bortolin M, Vassena C, Taschieri S, Del Fabro M. Antimicrobial activity of pure platelet-rich plasma against microorganisms isolated from oral cavity. *BMC Microbiol.* 2013; **13**:47.
30. Bielecki TM, Gazdzik TS, Arendt J, Szczepanski T, Krol W, Wielkoszynski T. Antibacterial effect of autologous platelet gel enriched with growth factors and other active substances: an in vitro study. *J Bone Joint Surg Br.* 2007;**89**:417-420.

31. Takakura N, Yoshida H, Kunisada T, Nishikawa S, Nishikawa S-I. Involvement of platelet-derived growth factor receptor-alpha in hair canal formation. *J Invest Dermatol*. 1996;**107**:770-7.
32. Saxena K, Saxena DK, Savant SS. Successful hair transplant outcome in cicatricial lichen planus of the scalp by combining scalp and beard hair along with platelet rich plasma. *J Cutan Aesthet Surg* 2016;**9**:51-5. doi: 10.4103/0974-2077.178562
33. Stojadinovic O, Morrison B, Tosti A. Adverse effects of platelet-rich plasma and microneedling. *J Am Acad Dermatol* 2020;**82**:501-2.
34. Latalski M, Walczyk A, Fatyga M, Rutz E, Szponder T, Bielecki T, et al. Allergic reaction to platelet-rich plasma (PRP): case report. *Medicine (Baltimore)*. 2019;**98**:e14702. doi:10.1097/MD.0000000000014702.
35. Kalyam K, Kavoussi SC, Ehrlich M, Teng CC, Chadha N, Khodadadeh S, et al. Irreversible blindness following periocular autologous platelet-rich plasma skin rejuvenation treatment. *Ophthalmic Plast Reconstr Surg*. 2017;**33**:S12-S16.
36. Owczarczyk-Saczonek A, Wygonowska E, Budkiewicz M, Placek W. Serum sickness disease in a patient with alopecia areata and Meniere' disease after PRP procedure. *Dermatol Ther*. 2019;**32**:e12798.
37. Garg S, Bansal A. Platelet-rich plasma in interventional dermatology and trichology: how far have we come? *Cosmoderma* 2021;**1**:12.
38. Garg S, Pandya I, Bhatt S. Follicular unit extraction (FUE) hair transplantation in combination with platelet rich plasma for the treatment of scarring alopecia: a case series. *Arch Clin Med Case Rep*. 2019;**3**:299-308.

CHAPTER 7

PLATELET-RICH PLASMA AND ITS USE IN HAIR DISORDERS IN COVID TIMES

RUBINA ALVES

Platelet-rich plasma (PRP) is a biological product defined as a portion of the plasma fraction of autologous blood with a platelet concentration above the baseline.[1] Besides the high level of platelets, PRP contains a full complement of clotting factors,[2] the latter typically remaining at their normal, physiologic levels.[3] It is also enriched by a range of growth factors (GFs), chemokines, cytokines and other plasma proteins.[3]

Platelet-rich plasma is currently used in different medical fields. The interest in the application of PRP in dermatology has recently increased, especially in the area of hair disorders.

Regarding hair diseases, PRP was mostly used and studied in patients presenting with androgenetic alopecia (AGA). Although there are several treatment options available for the treatment of patterned hair loss, currently, only topical minoxidil and oral finasteride have received the approval of the Food and Drug Administration (FDA) for the treatment of AGA.[4]

PRP has now emerged as a new potential therapeutic tool for hair loss disorders, both in non-cicatricial alopecia (androgenetic alopecia and telogen effluvium) and cicatricial alopecia (lichen planopilaris, frontal fibrosing alopecia, folliculitis decalvans).

Gupta AK et al.[5] performed a meta-analysis with the main objective to assess the effectiveness of PRP as a treatment for AGA. Ten studies,[1,6-14] whose parameters were considered more scientifically rigorous, were selected and the results of this meta-analysis favour the treatment of PRP when compared with placebo and baseline.

Most of the published articles describe the use of PRP alone but in our clinical practice, most of the patients are under several medical treatments. So, should we consider adding PRP to the medical treatment or should we also consider it as a monotherapy?

The results of a randomized placebo-controlled, double-blind, half-head study[1] to assess the efficacy of platelet-rich plasma on the treatment of AGA revealed that the administration of PRP as monotherapy led to a statistically significant increase in the mean anagen hairs, telogen hairs, hair density and terminal hair density after three months and after six months when compared with baseline.

In the second study,[15] it was hypothesized that PRP could lead to hair regrowth if used in combination with the patient's current medication. A randomized placebo-controlled, double-blinded, half-head study to assess the efficacy of PRP in combination with minoxidil or finasteride in the treatment of AGA was performed. The authors defined two groups of treatment: Group A included patients who received treatment with PRP plus oral finasteride on half-head and placebo on the other half, while Group B included patients who received treatment with PRP along with 5% topical minoxidil solution on half-head and placebo on the other half. Based on the results of the study, it was demonstrated that the administration of PRP in combination with medication is effective in AGA, statistically improving the mean hair parameters between six months and baseline. Both minoxidil and finasteride in combination with injections of PRP improved hair regrowth, although PRP in combination with minoxidil showed a greater improvement than PRP with finasteride, at six months.

New findings[16] also suggest that the hair growth-promoting effect of other biologic therapies, hair inductive drugs or surgical techniques can be significantly improved by adding PRP.

The treatment of androgenetic alopecia should be initiated as early as possible as untreated androgen-dependent alopecia progressively deteriorates.[17] Regarding AGA, at least three cycles of injections of PRP are necessary to achieve increased hair density and new hair regrowth. Patients should repeat treatment every six months to maintain the obtained results.

Telogen effluvium

Telogen effluvium (TE) is a non-scarring, diffuse hair loss from the scalp that occurs within three months after a triggering event and is usually self-limiting, lasting for about six months. It is a heterogeneous entity with numerous possible triggers such as metabolic or nutritional alterations, fever or medications.[18]

The COVID-19 pandemic has affected more than 125 million people worldwide and continues to spread across the globe. A large number of cutaneous manifestations have also been reported after a SARS-CoV-2 infection. Some hair disorders, such as alopecia areata and androgenetic alopecia were demonstrated to be associated with COVID-19, although acute TE appears to be the most common.[19]

In this pandemic area, several articles[18-22] have reported the association between SARS-CoV-2 infection and the increased number of cases of telogen effluvium. Moreno-Arrones et al.[18] hypothesize that in the case of SARS-CoV-2 associated TE, pro-inflammatory cytokines released during the infection can induce an immediate anagen release of the hair follicles, which switch to the catagen phase and subsequently enter telogen.

As mentioned by the authors, the data obtained from these patients suggests that a symptomatic SARS-CoV-2 infection is a risk factor for the development of acute TE. So, a past SARS-CoV-2 infection should be considered in every patient consulting for acute TE. Usually, it can develop after four weeks (early onset) or twelve weeks (late onset) from the time of infection. In addition, as the information regarding the time of onset and severity is similar to other infection-induced acute TE, it could be expected that the evolution and prognosis are similar and even without any specific treatment, full recovery of lost hair may occur.[18]

But in some of these patients the hair shedding is severe, and a precocious treatment is recommended. In selected cases, platelet-rich plasma might be considered a therapeutic option.

In a published study among patients with COVID-19 infection, confirmed using polymerase chain reaction (PCR) testing, PRP of the scalp was performed.

The authors reported that at the end of the first session, a 25%–54% reduction in hair loss was achieved in all patients according to the hair pull test.[23]

According to my experience, patients with telogen effluvium (with different causes such as pregnancy or post-SARS-CoV-2 infection) benefit from PRP injections as it significantly diminishes the shedding observed and helps to increase the density and hair regrowth. After only two cycles of PRP injections at the one-month intervals, the patient can start to see the results with a decrease in the shedding of hair. (Figure 1)

Cicatricial alopecia

Cicatricial or scarring alopecia is usually a source of frustration for both the physician and the patient. Some conditions destroy the hair follicle and produce a scar. Other conditions produce permanent alopecia without scarring.[24] Recently, new observations point to the possible efficacy of PRP in conditions presenting with cicatricial alopecia such as lichen planopilaris (LPP),[24-28] frontal fibrosing alopecia (FFA)[24,29] and folliculitis decalvans (FD),[24,30] although a paucity of literature exists in this regard.

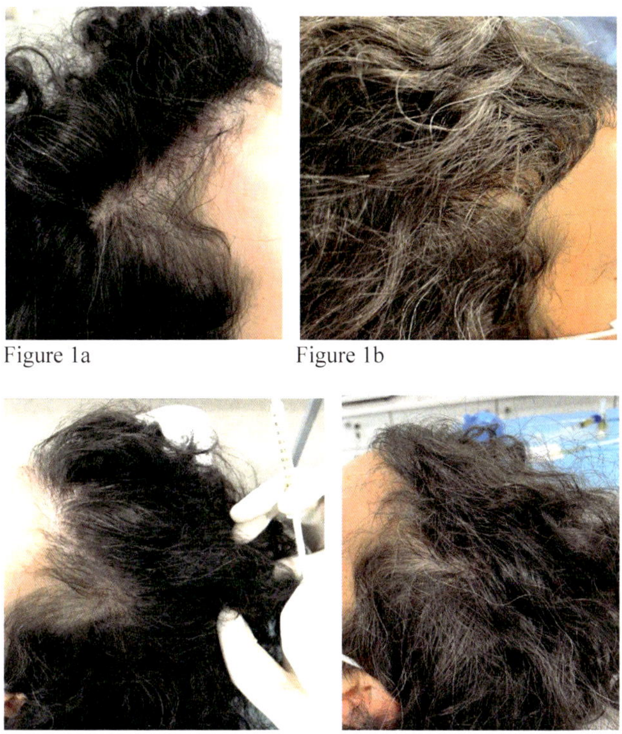

Figure 1a Figure 1b

Figure 1c Figure 1d

Figure 1: Female patient with acute telogen effluvium. Two sessions of PRP on monotherapy in the affected areas were performed. Figure 1a; Figure 1c: baseline; Figures 1b, 1d: after two sessions of PRP.

Lichen planopilaris

Lichen planopilaris is classified as a primary lymphocytic cicatricial alopecia and is difficult to treat. LPP frequently presents with hair loss at the vertex or parietal scalp and patients commonly experience associated scalp itching, burning or tenderness. The hair loss is typically permanent, and the treatment usually focuses on reducing symptoms and preventing disease progression.[25,26] Several articles[25-28] included clinical cases of patients diagnosed with LPP that were refractory to the other treatments. The patients were treated with three or four cycles of PRP and an increase in normal hair density across the scalp and frontal hairline with only minimal residual perifollicular erythema and scaling was reported.[26] Additionally, PRP was demonstrated to be effective in improving hair thickening and can be used as an adjunctive treatment along with topical minoxidil.[28]

My experience is similar to the findings mentioned above. It is usually necessary to perform at least three treatments of PRP (one month apart) to see the increase in hair density, hair thickness and absence of perifollicular inflammation. Also, patients report that the use of PRP diminishes the scalp itching and burning sensation. (Figure 2)

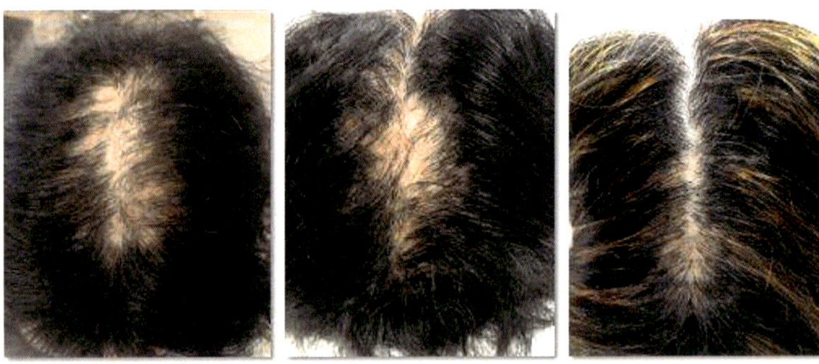

Figure 2a Figure 2b Figure 2c

Figure 2: Female patient with a diagnosis of lichen planopilaris. The patient performed three sessions with pure-PRP as monotherapy, injected in the affected areas (5 ml). After six months, there was an increase in hair density and regression of itching. Figure 7.2.a: baseline; Figure 7.2b: three months; Figure 7.3c: six months.

Frontal fibrosing alopecia

Frontal fibrosing alopecia (FFA) is currently the most frequent cicatricial alopecia. It is characterized by progressive recession of the frontal and temporoparietal hairline. It can also affect the eyebrows, eyelashes and body hair.[24]

Özcan et al.[29] described a case report of a 44-year-old female patient with FFA who performed several treatments such as 0.05% clobetasol propionate, oral hydroxychloroquine, topical 5% minoxidil lotion and injectable triamcinolone acetonide. The patient was refractory to the treatments, with continuous recession of the frontotemporal hairline, absence of hair regrowth on the eyebrows and persistence of clinical signs. The authors performed five sessions of PRP, injected into the frontotemporal hairline and eyebrows of the patient. After one month, there was an improvement in the perifollicular erythema, scaling and lichenoid papules on the frontotemporal hairline. There was a stabilization of the hair loss after five months.

In my clinical practice in the last few years, I have been performing PRP treatments in patients with FFA, especially in patients with persistent perifollicular inflammation, refractory to instituted treatments. As noted, at least five treatment sessions may be necessary to stabilize the follicular inflammation (Figure 3).

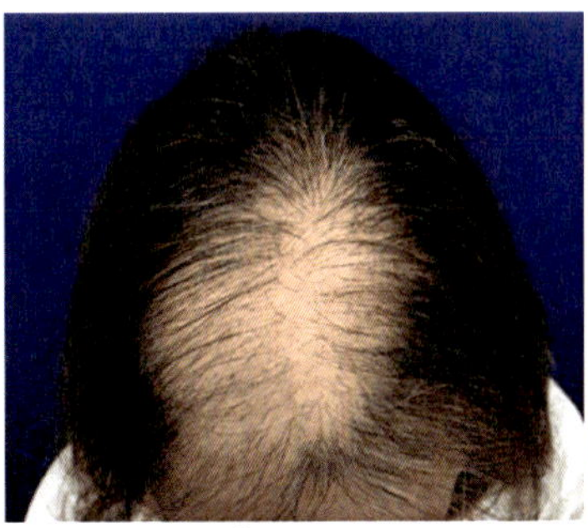

Figure 3a

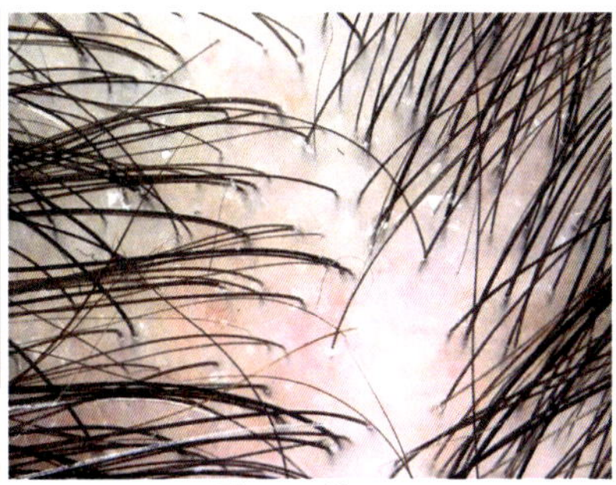

Figure 3b

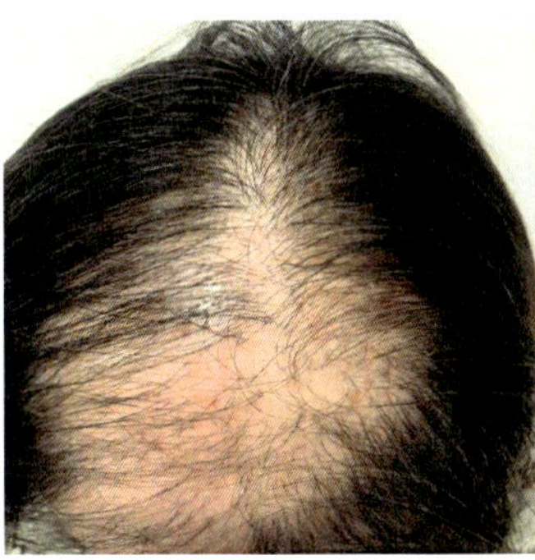

Figure 3c

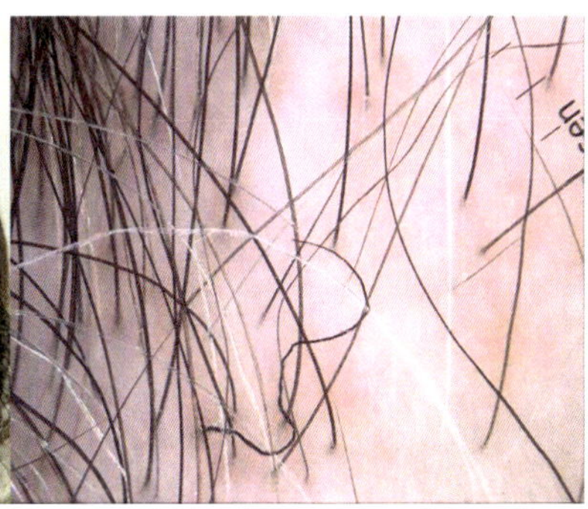

Figure 3d

Figure 3: Female patient with FFA in a pattern distribution, confirmed by skin biopsy. The patient was refractory to the treatment with the maintenance of perifollicular inflammation. After four sessions of PRP in the affected areas, there was a diminishing of the inflammation. The results were maintained after twelve months of follow-up.

Folliculitis decalvans

Folliculitis decalvans is a type of scarring alopecia which usually presents with tufted hair in the affected areas of the scalp, scaling and perifollicular pustules. It may be associated with pruritus or pain in the affected areas. Most of the treatments are unsatisfactory and do not lead to a full resolution of the disease.[24]

Shu et al.[30] described two patients with refractory FD. Four treatments with PRP, one month apart, were performed and after a single PRP treatment, significant improvement of the inflammation in both patients was noted. Patients experienced stability in hair loss and significant symptomatic improvement in inflammation with the subsequent PRP treatments. Although there was an improvement during the treatments, patients reported disease flares within four to five weeks following the last session of PRP. According to the authors, the positive effect of PRP was temporary and continued cycles of PRP treatments were necessary to maintain disease stability.

The reason why PRP might be useful in cicatricial alopecia is unknown. One of the hypotheses could be that various GFs would help diminish the inflammation, protecting and stimulating the new hair follicle. In addition, anti-inflammatory and pro-angiogenic cytokines that are present in the platelet granules may contribute to the effectiveness of PRP in cicatricial alopecias.[26]

Protocol of treatment

PRP is produced using different methods of platelet concentration via centrifugation and cell separation. There are several commercially available systems worldwide, with different characteristics that are defined by the manufacturer.

I personally recommend a closed system (the majority) that includes disposable kits and all the material necessary to prepare PRP. The PRP systems and equipment used for separation, concentration and plasma collection must meet all the applicable quality control criteria.

There is no standardized protocol worldwide regarding the use of PRP in hair disorders.

In my experience and considering the randomized studies[1,15] to assess the efficacy of platelet-rich plasma in the treatment of AGA, we should perform at least three cycles of PRP, one month apart.

After blood collection by venipuncture, the PRP is obtained according to the manufacturer's instructions (speed, centrifugation time, preparation method).

Then, we apply ice to the area to be treated, which is done 10 minutes before and during the injections. In the affected areas, PRP infiltration is performed with a 30 G needle at the dermal level and 0.15 ml–0.20 ml of PRP is injected proximally. Initially, at least three treatments with PRP (one month apart) should be performed. After six months, it is recommended to perform another three cycles of PRP for continued benefit and depending on the type of alopecia, more sessions may be needed. As for maintenance, it is important to perform treatments every six months or three cycles of PRP per year.

Contraindications for the treatment with PRP are fever, coagulation disorders, platelet abnormalities, systemic or scalp tumours, pregnancy and breastfeeding.[31]

There are a number of factors that could explain the variation obtained in PRP results.[5] Differences in preparations and delivery have been suggested as a possible explanation.[32,33] Monthly PRP injections had a significantly greater increase in hair count compared to injections every three months.[34] In addition, substantial improvements in hair restoration parameters (e.g. hair density, hair count) have frequently been reported in PRP studies that administer three monthly sessions, suggesting that three sessions may be necessary to achieve the desired results.[1,34]

Rodrigues et al.[35] performed a study where they analysed the platelet number and growth factor levels in PRP and the correlation with hair growth parameters three months before and after the last injection. The 26 patients received four subcutaneous injections and growth factors such as the platelet-derived growth factor (PDGF), the epidermal growth factor (EGF) and the vascular endothelial growth factor (VEGF), which were measured using a Luminex® method. The authors found a significant increase in hair count, hair density and percentage of anagen hairs in the PRP group when compared to the control group, although there was no correlation between platelet count or quantification of the growth factors in PRP. The authors proposed that other GFs not measured in their study may have been involved in the positive response seen with PRP.

There is also an intense ongoing debate regarding the ideal volume of PRP to administer, the frequency of application, the exact site of administration of PRP and which technique and preparation system of manufacture to use.[3] It would also be valuable to investigate the relationship between different concentrations of growth factors in PRP and the clinical outcomes as a paucity of literature exists in that regard.

A new multicentric study is being performed to quantify the number of platelets in each patient before centrifugation, and analyse the final concentration of platelets per injection (considering the total volume injected). The results of this study will help us to understand if there is an association between the doses injected and the results obtained in each patient.

Conclusion

The data analysed from different studies suggest that PRP has a beneficial role in hair regrowth although the frequency of treatments for effective results, and optimal duration of the therapy to maintain the results, is still unknown. When considering the use of PRP, although there are positive results with monotherapy, the use of PRP is more effective in combination with other medical treatments.

Initially, PRP was widely studied in patients with AGA where a favourable effect was demonstrated after injection therapy with PRP. Besides AGA, PRP is now being considered as a useful treatment option in telogen effluvium as it diminishes the associated shedding and accelerates the initiation of a new hair cycle.

PRP may be beneficial in selected patients with cicatricial alopecia, although the exact mechanism of action remains largely unknown. It is stated that the different GFs present in PRP could diminish the inflammation, protecting and stimulating the new hair follicle. PRP is a safe and effective treatment option for various hair disorders.

Further large-scale studies will help better understand the underlying mechanisms of PRP among the different hair disorders and fully utilize this tool to obtain the best result for each patient.

References

1. Alves R, Grimalt R. A randomized placebo-controlled, double-blind, half-head study to assess the efficacy of platelet-rich plasma on the treatment of androgenetic alopecia. *Dermatol Surg* 2016;**42**:491-497.
2. Wroblewski AP, Melia HA, Wright VJ. Application of platelet-rich plasma to enhance tissue repair. *Oper Tech Orthop* 2010;**20**:98-105.
3. Alves R, Grimalt R. A review of platelet-rich plasma: history, biology, mechanism of action, and classification. *Skin Appendage Disord.* 2018;**4**:18-24.
4. Alves R. Androgenetic alopecia: a review and emerging treatments. *Clin Res Dermatol Open Access* 2017;**4**:1-13.

5. Gupta AK, Cole J, Deutsch DP, Everts PA, Niedbalski RP, Panchaprateep R, et al. Platelet-rich plasma as a treatment for androgenetic alopecia. *Dermatol Surg*. 2019 Mar 11;**45**:1262-1273.
6. Anitua E, Pino A, Martinez N, Orive G, Berridi D. The effect of plasma rich in growth factors on pattern hair loss: a pilot study. *Dermatol Surg*. 2017;**43**:658-70.
7. Ayatollahi A, Hosseini H, Shahdi M, Ahmad Nasrollahi S, Yadangi S, et al. Platelet-rich plasma by single spin process in male pattern androgenetic alopecia: is it an effective treatment? *Indian Dermatol Online J*. 2017;**8**: 460-4.
8. Borhan R, Gasnier C, Reygagne P. Autologous platelet rich plasma as a treatment of male androgenetic alopecia: study of 14 cases. *J Clin Exp Dermatol Res*. Andhra Pradesh (India): OMICS; 2015. [No updated date; cited 26 January 2016] [Internet]. Available from: org/open-access/autologous-platelet-rich-plasma-as-a-treatment-of-male-androgenetic-alopecia-study-of-14-cases-2155-9554-10000292.php? aid=57866.
9. Cervelli V, Garcovich S, Bielli A, Cervelli G, Curcio MG, Orlandi A, et al. The effect of autologous activated platelet rich plasma (AA-PRP) injection on pattern hair loss: clinical and histomorphometric evaluation. *Biomed Res Int*. 2014;**2014**:760709.
10. Gentile P, Cole JP, Cole MA, Garcovich S, Bielli A, Scioli MG, et al. Evaluation of not-activated and activated PRP in hair loss treatment: role of growth factor and cytokine concentrations obtained by different collection systems. *Int J Mol Sci* 2017;**18**:PMC5343942.
11. Gentile P, Garcovich S, Scioli MG, Bielli A, Orlandi A, Cervelli V. Mechanical and controlled PRP injections in patients affected by androgenetic alopecia. *J Vis Exp* 2018; 2018. doi: 10.3791/56406.
12. Gkini M-A, Kouskoukis A-E, Tripsianis G, Rigopoulos D, Kouskoukis K. Study of platelet-rich plasma injections in the treatment of androgenetic alopecia through a one-year period. *J Cutan Aesthet Surg*. 2014;**7**:213-9.
13. Stevens HP, Donners S, de Bruijn J. Introducing platelet-rich stroma: platelet-rich plasma (PRP) and stromal vascular fraction (SVF) combined for the treatment of androgenetic alopecia. *Aesthet Surg J* 2018;**38**:811-22.
14. Takikawa M, Nakamura Shinichiro, Nakamura Shingo, Ishirara M, Kishimoto S, Sasaki K, et al. Enhanced effect of platelet-rich plasma containing a new carrier on hair growth. *Dermatol Surg* 2011;**37**:1721-9.

15. Alves R, Grimalt R. Platelet-rich plasma in combination with 5% minoxidil topical solution and 1 mg oral finasteride for the treatment of androgenetic alopecia: a randomized placebo-controlled, double-blind, half-head study. *Dermatol Surg*. 2018 Jan;**44**:126-130.
16. Anitua E, Pino A, Jaen P, Navarro MR. Platelet rich plasma for the management of hair loss: better alone or in combination? *J Cosmet Dermatol*. 2019;**18**:483-486.
17. Rushton DH, Ramsay ID, Norris MJ, Gilkes JJ. Natural progression of male pattern baldness in young men. *Clin Exp Dermatol*. 1991;**16**:188-192.
18. Moreno-Arrones OM, Lobato-Berezo A, Gomez-Zubiaur A, Arias-Santiago S, Saceda-Corralo D, Bernardez-Guerra C, et al. SARS-CoV-2-induced telogen effluvium: a multicentric study. *J Eur Acad Dermatol Venereol*. 2021;**35**:e181-e183. doi:10.1111/jdv.17045.
19. Starace M, Iorizzo M, Sechi A, Alessandrini AM, Carpanese M, Bruni F, et al. Trichodynia and telogen effluvium in COVID-19 patients: Results of an international expert opinion survey on diagnosis and management. *JAAD Int*. 2021;**5**:11-18.
20. Rossi A, Magri F, Sernicola A, Michelina S, Caro G, Muscianese M, et al. Telogen effluvium after sars-cov-2 infection: a series of cases and possible pathogenetic mechanisms. *Skin Appendage Disord*. 2021;**21**:1-5.
21. Monari P, Gualdi G, Bettoni G, Costa R, Ragni G, Zani F, et al. Post-SARS-CoV-2 Acute telogen effluvium: an expected complication. *J Clin Med*. 2022;**11**:1234.
22. Ocampo-Garza SS, Vastarella M, Nappa P, Cantelli M, Fabbrocini G. Telogen effluvium in the new SARS-CoV-2 era. *Int J Dermatol*. 2021;**60**:e265-e266.
23. Abrantes TF, Artounian KA, Falsey R, Simão JCL, Vañó-Galván S, Ferreira SB, et al. Time of onset and duration of post-COVID-19 acute telogen effluvium. *J Am Acad Dermatol*. 2021;**85**:975-976.
24. İşlek A, Karaaslan E, Şimşek S, Çetin FM. Platelet-rich plasma treatment for accelerated androgenetic alopecia pattern hair loss after COVID-19 infection: a case series. *J Cosmet Dermatol*. 2022 Feb;**21**:590-594.
25. Alves R, Grimalt R. Platelet-rich plasma and its use for cicatricial and non-cicatricial alopecias: a narrative review. *Dermatol Ther (Heidelb)*. 2020 Aug;**10**:623-633.
26. Svigos K, Yin L, Fried L, Sicco KL, Shapiro J. A practical approach to the diagnosis and management of classic lichen planopilaris. *Am J Clin Dermatol*. 2021 Sep;**22**:681-692.

27. Dina Y, Aguh C. Use of platelet-rich plasma in cicatricial alopecia. *Dermatol Surg*. 2019 Jul;**45**:979-981.
28. Jha AK. Platelet-rich plasma for the treatment of lichen planopilaris. *J Am Acad Dermatol*. 2018 Nov;79:e95-e96.
29. Jha AK. Platelet-rich plasma as an adjunctive treatment in lichen planopilaris. *J Am Acad Dermatol*. 2019 May;**80**:e109-e110.
30. Özcan D, Tunçer Vural A, Özen Ö. Platelet-rich plasma for treatment resistant frontal fibrosing alopecia: a case report. *Dermatol Ther*. 2019 Aug 23;**32**:e13072.
31. Suh S, Nguyen C, Zhao L, Mesinkovska NA. The role of platelet-rich plasma therapy in refractory folliculitis decalvans. *JAAD Case Rep*. 2021 Apr 24;**12**:85-87.
32. Alves R. Protocol: PRP in alopecia. In Alves R, Grimalt R, editors. Clinical indications and treatment protocols with platelet-rich plasma in dermatology. Barcelona: Ediciones Mayo; 2016. p. 82-83.
33. Castillo TN, Pouliot MA, Kim HJ, Dragoo JL. Comparison of growth factor and platelet concentration from commercial platelet-rich plasma separation systems. *Am J Sports Med*. 2011;**39**:266-71.
34. Mazzocca AD, McCarthy MBR, Chowaniec DM, Cote MP, Romeo AA, Bradley JP, et al. Platelet-rich plasma differs according to preparation method and human variability. *J Bone Joint Surg Am*. 2012;**94**:308-16.
35. Tawfik AA, Osman MAR. The effect of autologous activated platelet-rich plasma injection on female pattern hair loss: a randomized placebo-controlled study. *J Cosmet Dermatol* 2017;**17**:47-53.
36. Rodrigues BL, Montalvão SA, Cancela RB, Silva FA, Urban A, Huber SC, et al. Treatment of male pattern alopecia with platelet-rich plasma: a double-blind controlled study with analysis of platelet number and growth factor levels. *J Am Acad Dermatol*. 2018;**80**:694-700. doi: https://doi.org/10.1016/j.jaad.2018.09.033.

CHAPTER 8

THE ROLE OF PLATELET-RICH PLASMA THERAPY IN DIFFICULT-TO-TREAT SCARS

SHREYA AGGARWAL, ANUVA BANSAL, SURUCHI GARG, TRUSHA MISTRY

Introduction

A scar is a result of fibrosis due to chronic inflammatory changes occurring after the healing of a wound or ulcer. It presents clinically as an elevated or depressed area along with an alteration of skin texture, vascularity and nerve supply. Macroscopically, the anatomy of the skin is disturbed and there is a break in the continuity of normal skin. Microscopically, there is epidermal hypertrophy or atrophy, flattening of rete ridges and abnormal collagenization of the dermis. Though scars are considered trivial, they may be psychologically very disturbing and may affect the self-esteem of an individual, hence this should be addressed with the most appropriate treatment modality. Significant improvement has been demonstrated in various types of scars with the use of PRP. PRP enhances wound repair and tissue regeneration via the stimulation of collagen as well as elastin synthesis. It expedites healing and recovery, greatly reducing post-procedure downtime.

Pathogenesis of a scar

Following disruption of epithelial integrity, the process of scar formation is divided into three phases.

- The first 24–72 hours are an *inflammatory phase* where neutrophils are the main inflammatory cells.
- The next phase is the *proliferative phase* which is characterized by granulation tissue formation and macrophages releasing PDGF and

TGF, leading to collagen formation and angiogenesis. This phase typically lasts from 4 to 21 days.

- The last phase is that of *wound remodelling and contraction* which, if aberrant, can lead to hypertrophic scars. This is the longest phase in wound healing, lasting from 21 days to up to two years.

The arrangement of collagen during wound healing decides the type of scar formation (Table 1).

In normal scars, the collagen is small and in parallel bundles. Hypertrophic scars and keloids have thin and thick collagen fibres respectively, with increased collagen synthesis and cross-links.

Wound contraction is crucial as myofibroblasts contract to reduce the surface area of the scar.[1]

Table 1: Arrangement of collagen fibres and types of wounds

NATURE OF COLLAGEN					
	Orientation to epithelial surface	Bundle thickness	Synthesis	Collagen I/III ratio	Cross-links
Normal skin	Basketweave and parallel to epidermis	Normal	Normal	5:1	Normal
Scar	Fine, organized and parallel	Small	Increased	6:1	Less
Keloid	Haphazard and random	Large and thick	20 times	17:1	Double that of hypertrophic scar
Hypertrophic scar	Flat, wavy and parallel	Thin fibres arranged in nodular pattern	7 times	6:1	More

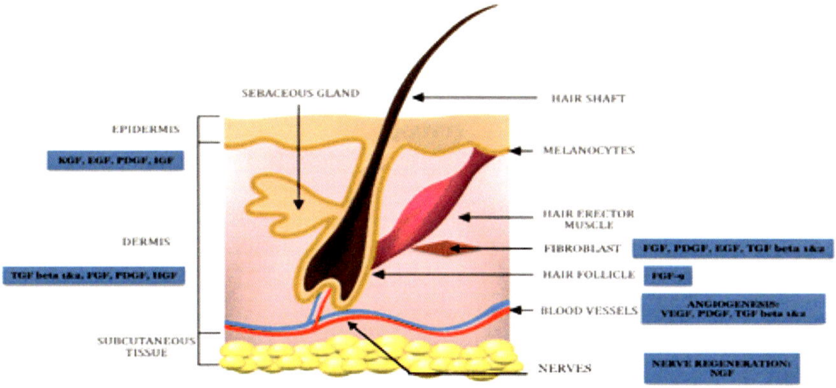

Figure 1: Normal anatomy of the skin and various growth factors in different tissues required for the wound healing process. PRP contains these growth factors in high concentration and aids in faster healing and improving the outcome.

Types of scars

Based on the underlying cause, scars can be post-traumatic, post-acne, post-surgical or post-burn scars.

Acne scars are further classified into atrophic (ice-pick, rolling, boxcar) and hypertrophic (papular, nodular, keloidal).

Various treatment modalities for scars

The treatment of scars is challenging because no single treatment is completely effective. Hence, multiple modalities have to be combined for good results.

The various treatment modalities in common practice are subcision, microneedling, punch excision, punch autograft, microdermabrasion, microneedling radiofrequency, sublative radiofrequency, phenol/trichloroacetic acid (TCA) peeling and lasers (CO_2 laser, erbium YAG laser, IPL, erbium glass, etc.), fat grafting, fillers, etc. It is imperative to understand the different types of scars and customize the treatment based on the morphology of individual scars. The advantage of using a cocktail of treatments is that different depths of scars are targeted, the total number of sessions is reduced, and the third regenerative component adds to the healing capacity of the treated area.

Why platelet-rich plasma therapy?

Platelet-rich plasma is an autologous concentrate of platelets suspended in small quantities of plasma. Various stimuli such as calcium chloride, thrombin and collagen cause platelet activation upon minimal induced injury.

The activated platelets release various growth factors such as platelet-derived growth factor (PDGF), insulin-like growth factor (IGF), vascular endothelial growth factor (VEGF), and platelet-derived angiogenic factor (PDAF), and transforming growth factor-beta (TGF-β) as demonstrated in Figure 1. These growth factors stimulate wound maturity and epithelialization, and thus limit scar tissue formation. The additional benefit of using cocktails helps in reducing the total number of sessions.

It also has a role in various regenerative processes such as epithelial differentiation, proliferation and angiogenesis. It improves microcirculation and collagen remodelling, and thus improves scar tissue texture.

As an adjuvant with autologous grafts, it helps improve the vascularity of the graft[2] and hence graft survival improves. Also, it helps other modalities such as lasers and fat grafts in better scar tissue remodelling.

The adjuvant PRP therapy helps in reducing the chances of post-inflammatory hyperpigmentation due to desiccating injuries by lasers and radiofrequency, and increases the healing process by supplying numerous growth factors over a period of time. Also, when combined with other modalities such as lasers and energy-based devices, it aids in faster healing of injuries induced by these modalities.

On the other hand, PRP can be used as an adjuvant to fat grafts for addressing the volume deficit and enhancing scar tissue remodelling.

Of late, the bio filler is gaining popularity as a temporary biocompatible replacement of fat grafts or fillers for correcting volume deficits. This is prepared by heating the harvested platelet-poor plasma followed by immediate cooling, leading to semisolid gel formation which can be injected through the cannula into the desired defect. The remaining platelet-rich plasma can still be injected over the skin for scar remodelling.

Role of platelet-rich plasma in scars

Platelet-rich plasma can be used as an effective adjuvant treatment modality as it hastens epidermal regeneration and collagen formation. (Box 1 and Table 2)

Various studies have been undertaken in recent times to demonstrate the effectiveness of platelet-rich plasma therapy in scar revision.

Box 1: Mechanism of action of PRP in scars

- increased proliferation of human dermal fibroblasts and stimulation of collagen synthesis;
- increased expression of matrix metalloproteinase (MMP) enhances the removal of photodamaged ECM;
- increased expression of G1 cell cycle regulators, accelerating wound healing;
- accelerated hyaluronic acid production, improved skin hydration;
- increased collagen type I via fibroblast stimulation;
- increased elastic fibres;
- new blood vessel formation;
- adipose tissue deposition;
- soft tissue augmentation.

Table 2: Mechanism of action, methods and outcomes of PRP in various types of scars

Indications	Mechanism of Action	Method	Results
Difficult Scars			
Atrophic acne scars Post-burn scars Post-traumatic scars Post-surgical scars	Increase in collagen type I via fibroblast stimulation Increase in elastic fibres New blood vessel formation Adipose tissue deposition Soft tissue augmentation	Microneedling and PRP injections Microneedling and topical PRP Laser and PRP injections Laser and topical PRP	Improvement in scar appearance – pigmentation, vascularity, skin texture Higher patient satisfaction Decreased post-procedural erythema and oedema Faster recovery, reduced downtime
Striae distensae	The thermal energy generated by bipolar radiofrequency (RF) denatures the elastic fibres and collagen bundles. PRP stimulates wound healing, thereby providing synergistic benefits and good results.	Intradermal RF device and PRP as a filler through its needle electrode PRP injection monotherapy PRP with ultrasound (Alma Impact)	Improves skin quality Increase in collagen and elastic fibres Reduced appearance of striae

Efficacy

Acne scars

Significant improvement in scars especially post-acne scars by the use of PRP alone, as well as in combination with microneedling or fractional ablative lasers, has been demonstrated. PRP augments wound repair and tissue regeneration via the stimulation of collagen as well as elastin synthesis. It expedites healing and recovery, thus greatly reducing the post-procedure downtime.

Gawdat et al.[3] compared fractional CO_2 laser alone with a fractional CO_2 laser with platelet-rich plasma in the treatment of atrophic acne scars. The results showed that patients treated with both modalities responded much better in terms of appearance, side effects and downtime compared to fractional CO_2 laser alone. This combination also reduced the post-procedure side effects, enhancing the overall patient experience with the added advantage of being painless.

Asif et al.[4] conducted a split-face study in 50 atrophic acne scar patients using combined microneedling and autologous platelet-rich plasma over the right half of the face, and microneedling alone over left half with 62.20% and 45.84% improvement respectively as per Goodman's quantitative scale. Redaelli et al.[5] conducted a study among 23 patients with acne scars over three months and concluded that PRP is a promising, easy to perform technique for scar attenuation. Fabbrocini et al.[6] conducted a study and found that PRP combined with microneedling was more effective in acne scars than microneedling alone. In a study on 30 patients with acne scars by Chawla et al.[7] It was concluded that PRP combined with microneedling is a better treatment option than microneedling with vitamin C.

Wounds and post-traumatic scars

In a review by Picard et al.,[8] a post-platelet-rich plasma clinical outcome was analysed in patients with acute wounds, post-laser therapies and burns. In the case of acute wounds, a statistically significant benefit was found in terms of healing time and pain. Platelet-rich plasma after laser therapies helped in faster wound healing and reducing erythema.

Carter et al.[9] studied equine wound healing after treating with platelet-rich plasma gel in terms of epithelial differentiation and regeneration. By day 7, there was intense cytokeratin staining of platelet-rich plasma treated wounds signifying faster epithelial regeneration and by day 79, dense and well-organized collagenization of the dermis was appreciated. They concluded that platelet-rich plasma leads to faster epithelial differentiation and improved collagen formation.

In a study on traumatic scars, Cervelli et al.[10] randomly divided 60 patients into three groups. The first group was treated with fat grafting and platelet-rich plasma, the second with non-ablative laser, and the third one with all of them. The third group showed the best results with 22% increase in wound healing compared to the first group. Gentile et al.[2] studied and compared the treatment response of stromal vascular factor enhanced autologous fat grafting (Group 1) and fat grafting with platelet-rich plasma (Group 2) in post-traumatic and burns scars. In Group 1, 63% of patients and in Group 2, 69% maintained the scar contour at the end of one year.

An in vitro pilot study[11] showed better fat graft volume, weight, vascularity and overall survival of the graft when mixed with platelet-rich plasma compared to that mixed with saline.

Striae Distensae *(SD)*

PRP acts by augmenting dermal elasticity via the stimulation of ECM and inducing synthesis of new collagen.[12]

A recent study compared the efficacy of PRP monotherapy, microdermabrasion (MD) and combination therapy with PRP and MD among 68 patients with SD. Significant clinical improvement was noted in those treated with PRP alone or PRP with MD when compared to MD alone, with no statistically significant difference in the outcomes between first two groups.[13] Studies comparing PRP monotherapy with topical tretinoin 0.05% cream applied once at night or tripolar radiofrequency found no statistically significant difference in the clinical outcome between the treatment groups.[14]

Carboxytherapy (CT) involves infusion of carbon dioxide gas via a subcutaneously placed needle. In a recent study comparing CT with PRP among 20 females with SD, significant clinical improvement was observed in all lesions, with no significant difference between treatment modalities.[15]

An intradermal radiofrequency (RF) device capable of delivering higher energy fluencies directly to the dermis is combined with injection of PRP through its needle electrode. Bipolar RF causes the denaturation of collagen and elastin fibres resulting in tissue contraction, while PRP stimulates neocollagenesis (NC) leading to tightening of the dermal tissue.[12] In a study among 19 patients with SD, this combination demonstrated marked improvement in majority of the cases.[16]

Very good or excellent improvement was seen at two months in the majority of the 18 women with striae alba treated with plasma fractional radiofrequency and enhanced PRP penetration, using acoustic wave ultrasound every two weeks for four sessions.[17]

PRP combined with the Pixel™ erbium YAG laser and microneedling radiofrequency (MNRF) treatment results in significant improvement in the erythema, pigmentation, skin texture and overall appearance in striae distensae, as observed by the author (Figure 2).

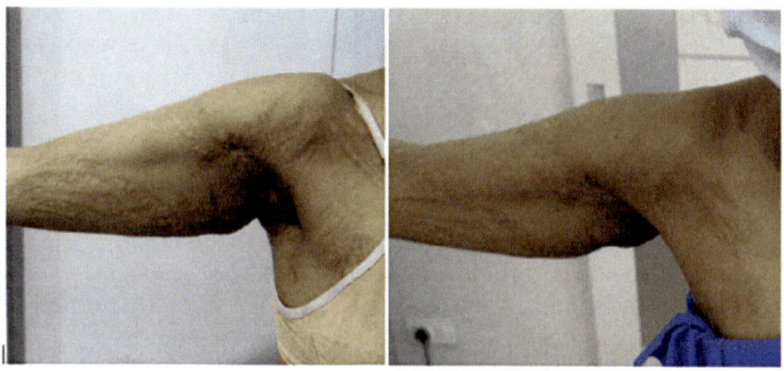

Figure 2: Improvement in striae distensae over the arms following three sessions of Pixel erbium YAG laser, MNRF and PRP therapy, in a 25-year-old patient with childhood onset nephrotic syndrome, undergoing corticosteroid therapy for a long duration (two years). Photo: Garg et al.[18]

Safety

Platelet-rich plasma therapy is autologous, hence no immunological or allergic side effects are anticipated. Local minor side effects such as pain or burning at the injection site, secondary infection or transient erythema can occasionally occur, which can be dealt with through adequate supportive care. It is always advisable to use a cannula while injecting large volumes or withdraw the plunger for at least 10–12 seconds while using a needle to avoid injecting into arteries.

Our experience

We commonly employ the use of PRP for difficult-to-treat scars as different cocktail treatments. These cocktails could be ablative lasers, microneedling radiofrequency along with PRP, or a combination of ablative and non-ablative lasers along with PRP and sometimes these combinations are used with fat grafting for adding volume to the subcutis.

We are sharing an interesting case where we used platelet-rich plasma therapy as an adjuvant to the Pixel erbium YAG laser and autologous fat grafting in a ***post-traumatic scar*** revision over the heel. This was a twenty-eight-year-old male patient who lost all sensations over the trauma site leading to repeated trophic ulcers. Our concept was to repeatedly ablate the scar tissue by erbium YAG laser followed by injections of platelet-rich plasma therapy for an effective wound repair. By the end of the third session, the patient started reporting appreciation of touch and pain sensations, which were completely absent at the start of surgery and were the principal cause of getting repeated trophic ulcers. The patient was given 15 ccs of autologous fat transplant beneath the heel subcutis in the fourth session along with the other two procedures. The fat was harvested from the medial side of the thigh under 2% injectable lignocaine solutions. By the end of five sessions, there was no trophic ulcer seen and the patient was extremely satisfied with the outcome overall; there was 40% improvement in touch and pain sensation on clinical examination. The second image in Figure 2 shows improvement after a four-month interval and the third one is after two and a half years of follow-up after an injury in the heel, which interestingly shows further improvement in the texture of skin and pigmentation, thus giving insight into ongoing work of PRP therapy and other combination modalities including fat grafting.

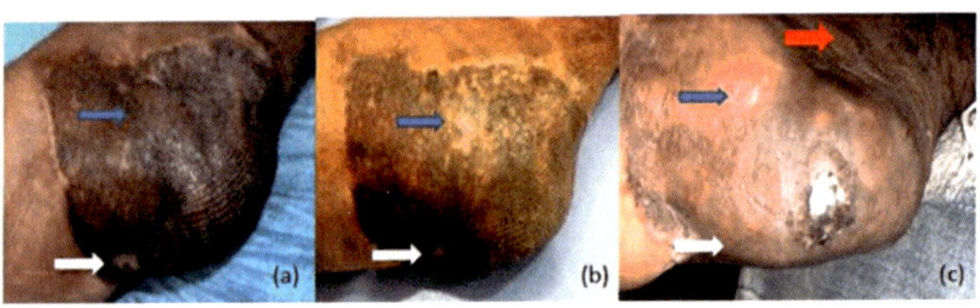

(a) Baseline photograph *(b) After 5 sessions of therapy* *(c) At the end of 2 ½ years following last session*

Figure 3: Post-traumatic scar with recurrent trophic ulcers due to lack of sensations after a pedicle graft over crushing heel injury. The scar was treated with a cocktail of Pixel erbium YAG laser, PRP therapy and autologous fat transplant. There is marked improvement in touch and pain sensation, texture, pigmentation of scar (blue arrows), healing of trophic ulcer (white arrows), and better merging of scar with surrounding skin (red arrows). Photo: Garg et al[19]

Figure 4 shows another post-traumatic scar treated with cocktail therapy.

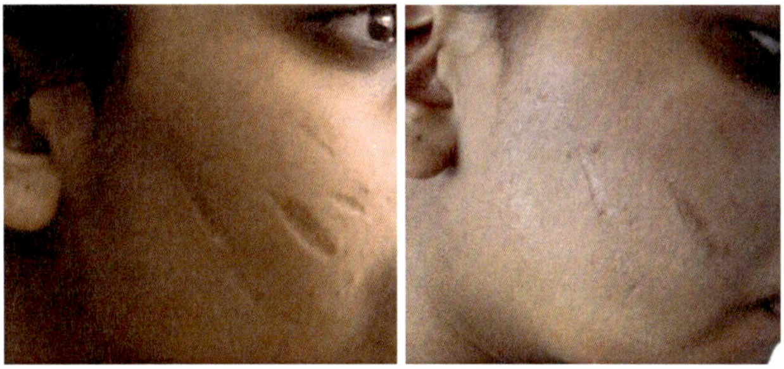

Figure 4: Post-traumatic scar treated with a cocktail treatment with three sessions of Pixel erbium YAG laser, microneedling radiofrequency and PRP. therapy. There is a perceptible reduction in number and depth of scars and an improvement in skin texture.

Post-acne atrophic scars: We find a combination of PRP therapy with Er:YAG laser resurfacing and microneedling radiofrequency to be an effective therapeutic modality for the treatment. This combination also helps in decreasing the downtime and incidence of adverse effects like post-inflammatory hyperpigmentation, which are conventionally associated with usage of Er:YAG lasers alone especially at higher fluence. Hence, more aggressive fluences can be used with less risk of post-inflammatory hyperpigmentation as is evident in Figures 4–6. The combination of different technologies also helps in addressing all three types of box car, rolling and ice-pick scars in fewer sessions.

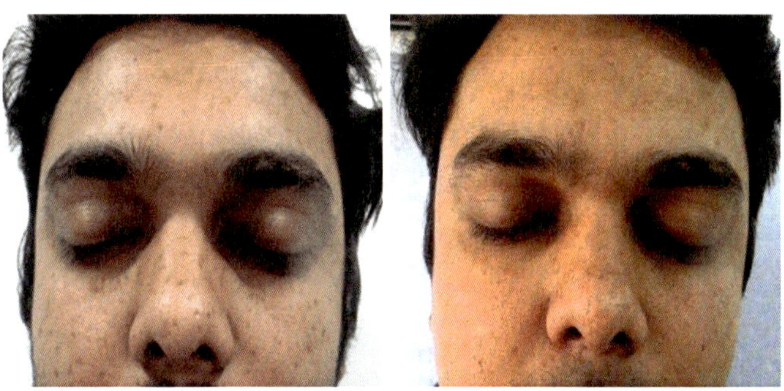

Figure 5: Post-acne and post chicken pox scars treated with two sessions of a cocktail of Pixel erbium YAG laser, microneedling radiofrequency and PRP therapy. There is uniform reduction in box car, rolling and ice-pick scars.

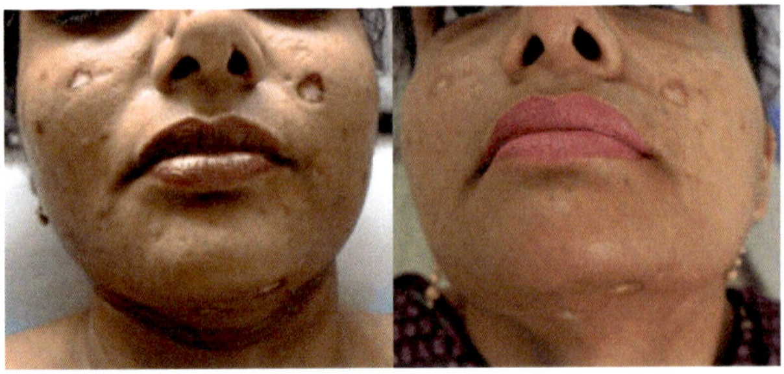

Figure 6: Post chicken pox scars presenting similar to DLE (discoid lupus erythematosus) scars after three sessions of a cocktail of PRP therapy, Pixel erbium YAG laser and microneedling radiofrequency. The patient was nutritionally depleted, with less than 50% of the daily recommended protein intake and underlying iron stores, vitamin D and B12 deficiencies. It is imperative to correct all these deficiencies beforehand, or the PRP growth signals and other therapeutic modalities may not be as effective, and the risk of post-inflammatory hyperpigmentation increases substantially. The de-pigmented patches may be treated along the lines of vitiligo management and may be considered for laser ablation and PRP-enriched epidermal suspension transplant in subsequent sessions.

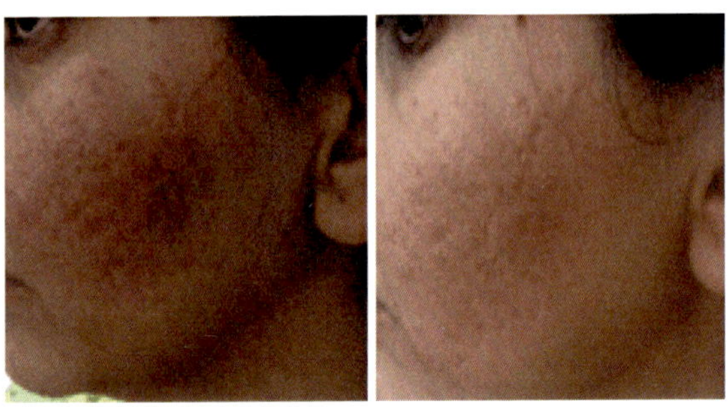

Figure 7: Post-acne scars after two sessions of a cocktail of Pixel erbium YAG laser, PRP therapy and microneedling radiofrequency. There is significant reduction in redness, boxcar, rolling and ice-pick scars; remaining linear scars should be discreetly targeted with ablative lasers in subsequent sessions.

More recently we have started other cocktails such as Alma Hybrid laser (CO_2 and 1570 nm) along with sublative radiofrequency. PRP therapy is infused through low-frequency ultrasound IMPACT^{TM} technology, which is a relatively painless infusion compared to injectable PRP therapy (Figure 8).

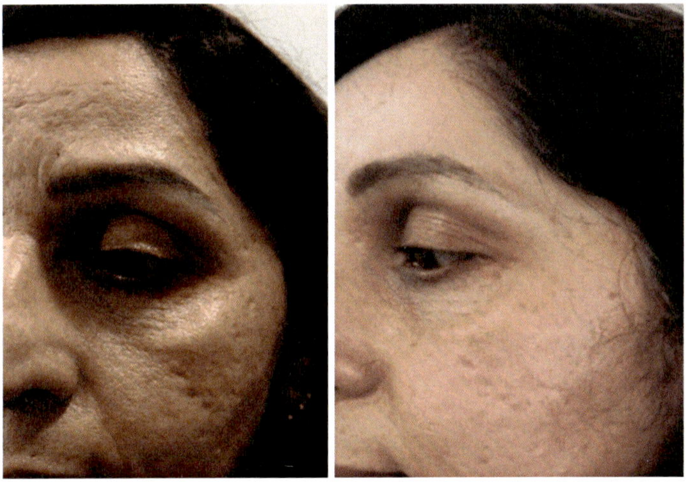

Figure 8: Post-acne scars and facial rejuvenation addressed with two sessions of a cocktail of Alma Hybrid laser (CO_2 with 1570 nm laser), sublative radiofrequency (forehead) along with PRP infusion through IMPACT^{TM}.

While PRP cocktails are yielding impressive results in difficult-to-treat scars, PRP also holds a promising role in hastening the recovery of an acute injury as shown in Figure 8. Infusion of high concentration of growth factors helps in rapid wound healing without sequelae.

Conclusion

Regenerative medicine, especially PRP therapy, is an easily accessible powerhouse of growth factors. When harvested and used in combination with cocktail treatments, it carries an immense scope for faster recovery, minimizing the number of sessions and side effects, and simultaneously improving the overall expected outcome. Another discreet advantage of adding PRP growth factors is that it apparently keeps on working in improving the tissue repair and regenerative process over subsequent years.

References

1. Bennett NT, Schultz GS. Growth factors and wound healing: biochemical properties of growth factors and their receptors. *Am J Surg*. 1993;**165**:728-37.
2. Gentile P, De Angelis B, Pasin M, Cervelli G, Curcio CB, Floris M, et al. Adipose-derived stromal vascular fraction cells and platelet-rich plasma: basic and clinical evaluation for cell-based therapies in patients with scars on the face. *J Craniofac Surg*. 2014;**25**:267-72.
3. Gawdat HI, Hegazy RA, Fawzy MM, Fathy M. Autologous platelet rich plasma: topical versus intradermal after fractional ablative carbon dioxide laser treatment of atrophic acne scars. *Dermatol Surg*. 2014;**40**:152-61.
4. Asif M, Kanodia S, Singh K. Combined autologous platelet-rich plasma with microneedling verses microneedling with distilled water in the treatment of atrophic acne scars: a concurrent split-face study. *J Cosmet Dermatol*. 2016;**15**:434-43.
5. Majid I. Microneedling therapy in atrophic facial scars: an objective assessment. *J Cutan Aesthet Surg*. 2009;**2**:26-30.
6. Fabbrocini G, De Vita V, Pastore F, Panariello L, Fardella N, Sepulveres R, et al. Combined use of skin needling and platelet-rich plasma in acne scarring treatment. *Cosmet Dermatol*. 2011;**24**:177-83.
7. Chawla S, Sacchidanand S, Leelavathi B. Split face comparative study of microneedling with PRP versus microneedling with vitamin C in treating atrophic post acne scars. *J Cutan Aesthet Surg*. 2014;**7**:209-212.
8. Picard F, Hersant B, Bosc R, Meningaud J-P. Should we use platelet-rich plasma as an adjunct therapy to treat "acute wounds," "burns," and "laser therapies": a review and a proposal of a quality criteria checklist for further studies. *Wound Repair Regen*. 2015;**23**:163-170.
9. Carter CA, Jolly DG, Worden CE Sr, Hendren DG, Kane CJM. Platelet-rich plasma gel promotes differentiation and regeneration during equine wound healing. *Exp Mol Pathol*. 2003;**74**:244-55.
10. Cervelli V, Nicoli F, Spallone D, Verardi S, Sorge R, Nicoli M, et al. Treatment of traumatic scars using fat grafts mixed with platelet-rich plasma, and resurfacing of skin with the 1540 nm nonablative laser. *Clin Exp Dermatol*. 2012;**37**:55-61.
11. Oh DS, Cheon YW, Jeon YR, Lew DH. Activated platelet-rich plasma improves fat graft survival in nude mice: a pilot study. *Dermatol Surg*. 2011;**37**:619-625.

12. Heitmiller K, Wang JV, Murgia RD, Saedi N. Utility of platelet-rich plasma for treatment of striae distensae: a current exploration. *J Cosmet Dermatol*. 2021 Feb;**20**:437-441.
13. Ibrahim ZAE-S, El-Tatawy RA, El-Samongy MA, Ali DAM. Comparison between the efficacy and safety of platelet-rich plasma vs. microdermabrasion in the treatment of striae distensae: clinical and histopathological study. *J Cosmet Dermatol.* 2015;**14**:336-346.
14. Gamil HD, Ibrahim SA, Ebrahim HM, Albalat W. Platelet-rich plasma versus tretinoin in treatment of striae distensae: a comparative study. *Dermatol Surg*. 2018;**44**:697-704.
15. Hodeib AA, Hassan GFR, Ragab MNM, Hasby EA. Clinical and immunohistochemical comparative study of the efficacy of carboxytherapy vs platelet-rich plasma in treatment of stretch marks. *J Cosmet Dermatol.* 2018;**17**:1008-1015.
16. Kim IS, Park KY, Kim BJ, Kim MN, Kim CW, Kim SE. Efficacy of intradermal radiofrequency combined with autologous platelet-rich plasma in striae distensae: a pilot study. *Int J Dermatol.* 2012;**51**:1253-1258.
17. Suh D-H, Lee S-J, Lee J-H, Kim H-J, Shin M-K, Song K-Y. Treatment of striae distensae combined enhanced penetration platelet-rich plasma and ultrasound after plasma fractional radiofrequency. *J Cosmet Laser Ther*. 2012;**14**:272-276.
18. Garg S, Bansal A. Platelet-rich plasma in interventional dermatology and trichology: how far have we come? *Cosmoderma* 2021;**1**:12.
19. Garg S, Saginathum S, Badheka A. Use of stem cells in intervention dermatology and trichology: a new hope. *J Stem Cell Res Dev Ther.* 2019;**5**:1-8.

CHAPTER 9

POST-BURN SCARS – FINALLY A HOPE

ANUVA BANSAL, SURUCHI GARG

Introduction

Burns refer to the tissue injury resulting from excessive thermal, chemical or electrical energy, primarily involving the skin and mucosa. These acute wounds resulting from an isolated traumatic event leading to cellular destruction, tend to heal through a series of stages and the healing process is largely dependent on the depth of the burn.[1,2,3]

First-degree burn wounds and the superficial second-degree burns heal faster, while the deep wounds show little tendency to heal spontaneously and are amenable to secondary infection.

Post-burn wound healing may lead to sequelae such as scar hyperplasia and contracture deformity, and prompt treatment of burns including debridement and infection prevention is paramount to effective healing. The extent of disfigurement and resistance to therapy have deemed post-burn scars as one of the most challenging scars to treat. The singeing and destruction of the underlying appendages, blood vessels and nerve tissue, besides the damage to the superficial layers, poses another difficulty.[1,4]

Current research suggests that PRP can significantly accelerate the healing process and result in improvement in the post-burn scar pigmentation, texture and associated neuropathic pain. In our experience, PRP should be considered as an important adjunct in the treatment of post-burn scars.[1,4,5]

Healing of burn wounds

a) Depth of burn wounds

The healing potential and need for surgical grafting is primarily dependent on the depth of the burn. Cutaneous burns are classified based on the depth of tissue injury as follows: (Table 1)

- In first-degree and second-degree superficial burns, healing occurs by primary intention.
- Second-degree superficial burns tend to heal without scarring in five to seven days and utilize the *epithelium of hair follicle* remnants present in the superficial dermis.
- In second-degree deep and third-degree burns, healing occurs by secondary intention, with epithelization and contraction.[6-8]

b) Pathophysiology of healing in burn wounds

The healing of burn wounds proceeds through the stages of inflammation including a vascular response and a cellular response. This is followed by the proliferative phase and the final stage of collagen matrix formation, resulting in maturation and remodelling into scar tissue. (Table 2).[9] Several cytokines and growth factors such as transforming growth factor-beta (TGF-β), platelet-derived growth factor (PDGF), vascular endothelial growth factor (VEGF) and basic fibroblast growth factor (bFGF) function to facilitate this transition from one phase to another.[4,6-9]

Disturbance and imbalance in this normal reparative process may result in various complications of healing in burn wounds, including scarring, contractures and pigmentary changes. (Table 3). Factors responsible for abnormal wound healing include malnutrition, vitamin D deficiency, vitamin C deficiency, diabetes, heart failure, smoking, radiation and wound infection, particularly with *Pseudomonas* and *Acinetobacter*.

Table 1: Depth of burn wounds[6-8]

Depth	Morphology	Sensation	Healing	Type of scar
Superficial (first-degree) (epidermal)	Dry, erythematous Blanches with pressure	Painful	Three to six days	No scarring
Superficial partial-thickness (second-degree superficial) (epidermis + superficial dermis)	Blisters Moist, red, weeping Blanches with pressure	Painful to temperature, air and touch	7 to 21 days	Scarring is unusual; pigment changes can occur
Deep partial-thickness (second-degree deep) (epidermis + deep dermis) can damage hair follicles and glands	Blisters Wet or waxy dry Variable mottled colour Blanching with pressure may be sluggish	Painful to pressure only	>21 days, (range: two to nine weeks) usually requires surgical treatment	Hypertrophic scarring If it fails to heal in two weeks it is functionally and cosmetically equivalent to a full-thickness burn.
Full-thickness (third-degree burn) (epidermis + dermis + subcutaneous tissue)	No blistering Waxy white to leathery grey to charred and black Dry and inelastic No blanching with pressure Hair can be pulled from follicles	Deep pressure only	Rare, unless surgically treated	Severe scarring Wound contracture with epithelialization around the wound edges
Deeper injury (i.e. fourth degree) Extends through the skin into underlying soft tissue and can involve muscle and/or bone.	Extends into fascia and/or muscle	Deep pressure	Never, unless surgically treated	Severe scarring, contracture

Adapted from Mertens et al.,[6] Peate,[7] and Clayton et al.[8]

Table 2: Phases of healing in burn wounds[9]

Phases of healing in burn wounds	
1. Inflammatory phase (reactive)	Immediately after the injury, the inflammatory response of the body begins, which has vascular and cellular components. *Vascular response*: local vasodilatation with fluid extravasation occurs immediately after burns. *Cellular response*: neutrophils and monocytes are the earliest cells to reach the site of inflammation. They are replaced later by macrophages, which phagocytose dead tissue and toxins released by the burned tissue.
2. Proliferative phase and formation of granulation tissue (reparative)	1. Migration of keratinocytes from viable skin appendages starts within a few hours after injury; re-epithelization is completed within five to seven days. 2. Basement membrane is formed. 3. Angiogenesis and fibrogenesis occur.
4. Collagen matrix formation and maturation (remodelling)	1. The laying down of collagen and elastin forms an extracellular matrix. 2. The extracellular matrix remodels into scar tissue. 3. Fibroblast transforms into myofibroblasts, resulting in scar contraction.

Table 3: Complications of wound healing in burns

Complications of wound healing in burns	Type of burn	Pathophysiology
• Hypertrophic scarring • Contractures	Second-degree deep dermal Full-thickness burns	Healing by secondary intention results in prolongation of resolution phase; it may take a year.
• Hyperpigmentation	Superficial burns	Overactive response of melanocytes to burn trauma occurs.
• Hypopigmentation	Deep burns	There is destruction of melanocytes of the skin appendages.
• Hyperpigmentation of graft in dark skin • Hypopigmentation of graft in white skin.	Grafted areas	Growing nerves alter the melanocyte control.

Mechanism of action of PRP in burn wounds and post-burn scars

The various growth factors (VEGF, TGF-β, bFGF, PDGF) and inflammatory mediators (chemokines and cytokines) released by PRP augment the impaired healing process in burn wounds, resulting in neovascularization (NV) and neocollagenesis (NC).[4] Recent research indicates that these growth factors promote cellular proliferation, differentiation and effective migration of epidermal keratinocytes, and promote wound healing. (Table 4)

PRP also leads to the release of certain nerve growth factors and neuroimmunophilin ligands, which can initiate nerve healing and regeneration, leading to improvement in sensations.[10] The plethora of growth factors, stem cell factors and leukotrienes released by PRP also function to restore hair follicle integrity, and may help regenerate the injured follicles.[11]

This platelet-rich concentrate functions to restore the balance between anti-inflammatory and pro-inflammatory stimuli by controlling the local inflammatory milieu, and tips the equilibrium in favour of inflammation resolution, resulting in effective healing.[12] Platelets have bactericidal and antibacterial effects, and can accelerate wound healing.[13]

Technique

In a study involving monthly sessions of PRP for a total of three sessions among 19 patients, 0.2–0.3 ml PRP was injected into the scar using a 3 ml syringe with a 30G needle utilizing the "linear retrograde and fanning" techniques, along with two or three retrograde injections known as "tunnelling", where a back-and-forth movement of the needle is applied to create a tunnel and a track, which is then loaded with the solution.

Significant improvement was observed in itching, pigmentation and pliability of scars. Improvement in pain was also experienced and may be attributed to nerve GFs, which help in nerve healing and regeneration.[14]

Various treatment combinations such as fat grafting, resurfacing of the skin using CO_2 or a 1540 nm non-ablative laser and PRP are associated with improvement in the post-burn scars.[15-17]

Our experience

PRP monotherapy with intralesional injections augments wound healing. (Figure 1)

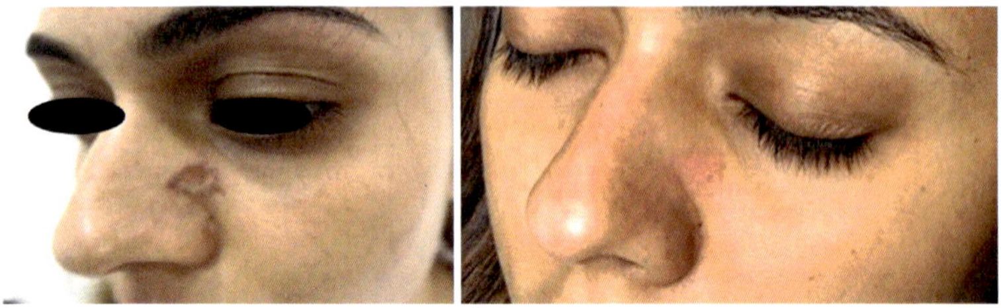

Figure 1: Acute cigarette burn showing good healing after five days of single-session PRP injection.

The authors have utilized a combination cocktail treatment consisting of PRP, an ablative Er:YAG Pixel™ laser and microneedling radiofrequency (MNRF) in five patients of post-burn scars.

Method

Microneedling radiofrequency (de-age: 3 mm depth at 35 mj output, three passes) was done first followed by instillation of platelet-rich plasma (.05 ml at a gap of 0.5 cm) each through insulin syringe and ablative laser (Alma lasers, Harmony platform; 1300 mj/p, five passes). Topical anaesthesia cream EMLA™ was applied for half an hour prior to the procedure. PRP was prepared using two Renew cell kits containing a total of 27 ml of whole blood with 3 cc of ACD-A as anticoagulant, centrifuged at 3200 RPM and 1350 RCG in a Remi cold centrifuge at 8–10 temperature, harvesting 5–6 ml of PRP with platelet concentration of 3–4 times the baseline value (average count nearly 10 lac). The sessions were repeated every three weeks for a total of three sessions (Figures 2 and 3).

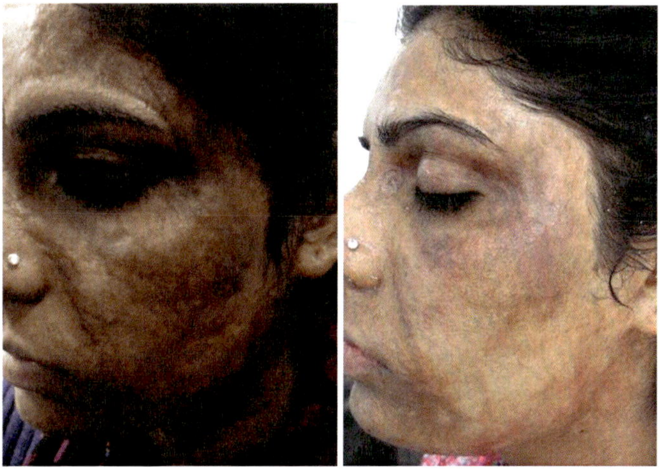

Figure 2: Post-burn scar treated with a cocktail of three sessions of Er:YAG Pixel laser, microneedling radiofrequency and PRP injections

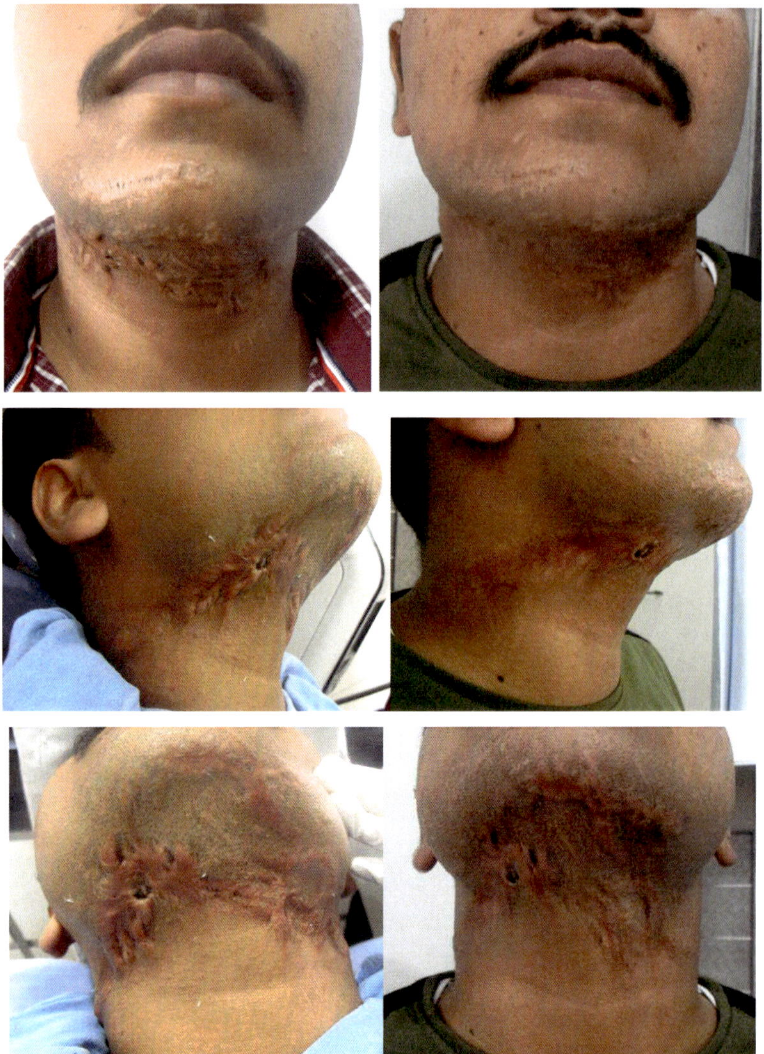

Figure 3: Post-burn scar treated with three sessions of cocktail of Er:YAG Pixel laser, microneedling radiofrequency and PRP therapy. There is significant improvement in contractures and thickened bands with improved range of neck extension.

Results

The scars were assessed using the POSAS (Patient and Observer Scar Assessment Scale). All patients were assessed for the improvement in pigmentation, vascularity, relief in terms of skin texture, thickness, pliability in a scale of 0–10 and for the appearance of hair follicles (yes/no). A maximum improvement of 3.8 points was noted within the mean values of pigmentation, while thickness and vascularity showed a difference of 1.4 points each in the mean value. The values obtained in the Patient Scar Assessment Scale based on the questionnaire are a maximum improvement of 4.2 points. It was seen in mean values of colour, while mean values of pain showed an improvement of 1.2 points. There was an appearance of new hair follicles noticed in 4 out of 5 patients (Figure 4).

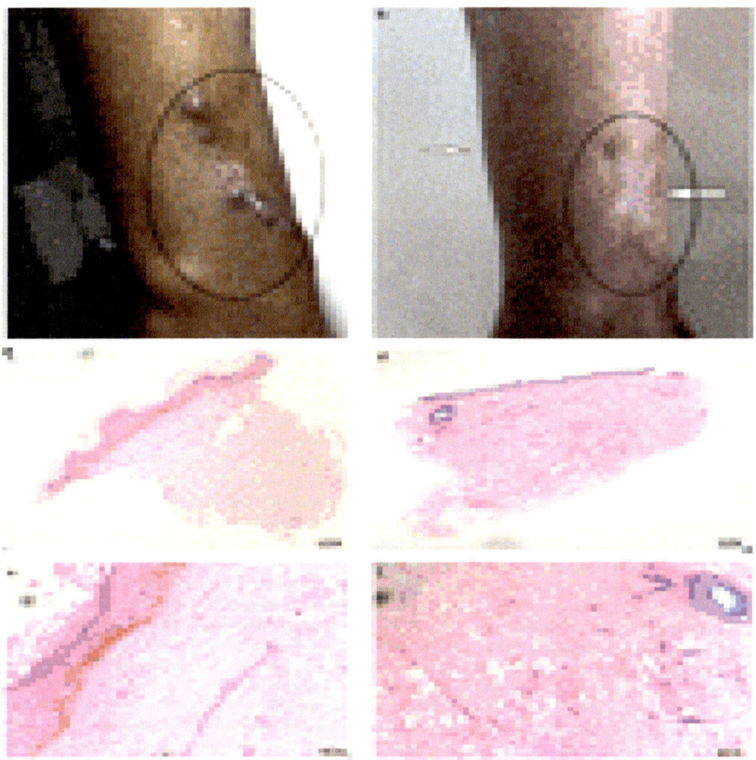

Figure 4: Post-burn scar revision a) before and b) after a cocktail treatment and regeneration of new hair follicle before 10× – c) and 40× – e) and after visible hair follicles in 10× – d) and 40× – f) histopathological images. Photo: SCRI[4].

Conclusion

These results were based on the principle of regenerative medicine where laser and MNRF help in resurfacing old, scarred skin, induce micro-injuries, activate dormant hair follicles and form new vessels, nerves and repair damaged appendages. It is trusting the body's own regenerative capacity further supported effectively by GFs, cytokines, chemokines and plasma proteins released by PRP.

Future directions

Post-burn scars result frequently in both functional and aesthetic severe impairments in restitution and rehabilitation periods of the burn disease.

Current research suggests that PRP can significantly accelerate the healing process and result in improvement in the post-burn scar pigmentation, texture and associated neuropathic pain. In our experience, PRP should be considered as an important adjunct in the treatment of post-burn scars.

Recent studies have demonstrated noteworthy improvements in post-burn scars following both autologous lipografting and mesenchymal stem cell application (MSC), as demonstrated by reduced Vancouver Scar Scale scores and clinical appearance, with clinical regression of the hypertrophic scars. Similar to growth factors released by PRP, MSCs are capable of promoting the renewal processes within a body, while having an effect not only on the processes of active transport, differentiation and entering into the damaged tissues, but also on promoting angiogenesis, and offering anti-inflammatory and anti-fibrotic properties. Lipofilling and adipose MSCs seem promising to lessen the severity of developing as pre-existent fibrotic scarring as well.[18]

Future biological, immunological and clinical research in the treatment of post-burn scars and chronic wounds with platelet-rich plasma derived growth factors and mesenchymal stem cells are warranted to augment post-burn wound healing and alleviate the resulting scars.

Table 4: Mechanism of action of PRP in burn wounds and post-burn scars[4, 10-13]

Mechanism of action	Method	Results	Outcome
• Increase in collagen type I via fibroblast stimulation • Increase in elastic fibres • Normalizing keratinocyte – melanocyte milieu by presence of fibroblast growth factor • New blood vessel formation • Adipose tissue deposition • Soft tissue augmentation • Hair follicle regeneration and survival • Initiation of nerve healing and regeneration • Restoration of the balance between anti-inflammatory and pro-inflammatory stimuli • Bactericidal and antibacterial effects	1. Microneedling and PRP injections 2. Microneedling and topical PRP 3. Laser and PRP injections 4. Laser and topical PRP	• Improvement in scar appearance: ○ pigmentation ○ vascularity ○ skin texture • Improved sensation and reduction in pain scores • Hair follicular growth	• Higher patient satisfaction • Decreased post-procedural erythema and oedema • Faster recovery, reduced downtime and infection rate

References

1. Hawkins HK, Pereira CT. Pathophysiology of the burn scar. In: Herndon DN, editor. Total burn care. 3rd edition. Philadelphia: Saunders Elsevier; 2007. p. 608-619.
2. Greenhalgh DG. Management of burns. *N Engl J Med* 2019;**380**:2349-59.
3. Huang H, Sun X, Zhao Y. Platelet-rich plasma for the treatment of burn wounds: a meta-analysis of randomized controlled trials. *Transfus Apher Sci*. 2021 Feb;**60**:102964.
4. Garg S, Badheka A, Singhal S. A pilot study of making new skin and appendages for post burn scars through a unique cocktail of platelet rich plasma, ablative Pixel Erbium:Yag laser and microneedling radiofrequency. *Stem Cell Res Int*. Kansas US: Opast Publishing; 2018. [no updated date; cited 19 April 2022] [Internet]. Available from: https://www.opastonline.com/wp-content/uploads/2018/11/a-pilot-study-of-making-new-skin-and-appendages-for-post-burn-scars-through-a-unique-cocktail-of-platelet-rich-plasma-ablative-pixel-erbium-yag-laser-and-micro-needling-radiofrequency-scri-18.pdf
5. Huang S-H, Wu S-H, Lee S-S, Lin Y-N, Chai C-Y, Lai C-S, et al. Platelet-rich plasma injection in burn scar areas alleviates neuropathic scar pain. *Int J Med Sci*. 2018;**15**:238-47.
6. Mertens DM, Jenkins ME, Warden GD. Outpatient burn management. *Nurs Clin North Am* 1997;**32**:343.
7. Peate WF. Outpatient management of burns. *Am Fam Physician* 1992;45:1321.
8. Clayton MC, Solem LD. No ice, no butter. Advice on management of burns for primary care physicians. *Postgrad Med*. 1995;**97**:151.
9. Tiwari VK. Burn wound: How it differs from other wounds? *Indian J Plast Surg*. 2012;**45**:364-73.
10. Nita AC, Orzan OA, Filipescu M, Jianu D. Fat graft, laser CO_2 and platelet-rich plasma synergy in scars treatment. *J Med Life*. 2013;**6**:430-433.
11. Garg S. Post-traumatic scar with repeated trophic ulcers treated with a cocktail of ablative pixel Erbium YAG laser, PRP therapy and autologous fat transplant – a novel case report of terminal nerve ending regeneration through regenerative surgery. *J Mol Genet Med*. 2017;**11**:303.
12. Bohren Y, Timbolschi DI, Muller A, Barrot M, Yalcin I, Salvat E. Platelet-rich plasma and cytokines in neuropathic pain: a narrative review and a clinical perspective. *Eur J Pain*. 2022 Jan;**26**:43-60.

13. Chen Z, Wu Y, Turxun N, Shen Y, Zhang X. Efficacy and safety of platelet-rich plasma in the treatment of severe burns: a protocol for systematic review and meta analysis. *Medicine*. 2020 Nov 6;**99**: e23001.
14. Elsayed M. Evaluation of the effect of platelet-rich plasma on post-burn scars. OAJS **5**. 16 Aug 2017 [no updated date; cited 15 March 2022] [Internet]. Available from: https://juniperpublishers.com/oajs/OAJS. MS.ID. 555660.php
15. Nita AC, Orzan OA, Filipescu M, Jianu D (2013) Fat graft, laser CO_2 and platelet-rich plasma synergy in scars treatment. *J Med Life*. 2013;**6**:430-433.
16. Cervelli V, Nicoli F, Spallone D, Verardi S, Sorge R, Nicoli M, et al. Treatment of traumatic scars using fat grafts mixed with platelet-rich plasma, and resurfacing of skin with the 1540 nm nonablative laser. *Clin Exp Dermatol.* 2012;**37**:55-61.
17. Cervelli V, Palla L, Pascali M, De Angelis B, Curcio BC, Gentile P. Autologous platelet-rich plasma mixed with purified fat graft in aesthetic plastic surgery. *Aesthetic Plast Surg*. 2009;**33**:716-21.
18. Zahorec P, Sarkozyova N, Ferancikova N, Bukovcan P, Danisovic L, Bohac M, et al. Autologous mesenchymal stem cells application in post-burn scars treatment: a preliminary study. *Cell Tissue Bank*. 2021 Mar;**22**:39-46.

CHAPTER 10

THE ROLE OF PLATELET-RICH PLASMA IN SKIN REJUVENATION

TRUSHA MISTRY, ANUVA BANSAL, SURUCHI GARG

Introduction

Platelet-rich plasma is an autologous concentration of platelets in a small volume of plasma. Its use in various surgical and medical fields is well established. PRP has been used in dermatology in recent years either alone or in combination with other modalities for various conditions such as androgenetic alopecia, scar remodelling, volume augmentation, fat grafting and skin rejuvenation.

Skin ageing

Ageing is a natural process. Dermal tissue mainly comprises collagen and elastin fibres; collagen constitutes 80% of the dry weight of the skin and provides tensile strength. Elastin, on the other hand, provides flexibility and resilience. It is known that there are two types of ageing – chronological ageing and photoaging. The latter term denotes the aggravated ageing process due to sun exposure.

Clinically chronological ageing is characterized by a normal geometric pattern, exaggerated expression lines and increased fragility of the skin. Histopathologically with ageing, the stratum corneum remains largely unchanged, the epidermis is thinned out and the dermo-epidermal junction appears flattened. There is a considerable decrease in dermal thickness and vascularity, as well as a reduction in the number and biosynthetic capacity of fibroblasts that results in delayed wound healing. With age, the fine dermal elastic fibres become coarser and then disappear.

Clinical manifestations of photo-aged skin include rhytides, pigmentary changes, and loss of skin tone and elasticity. Histopathology reveals elastosis, epidermal atrophy, and distinct alterations in collagen and elastin fibres. Furthermore, it has been found to be associated with a reduced level of hyaluronic acid.

Skin rejuvenation

Ageing is inevitable but maintaining a youthful appearance is a priority for many people nowadays. With the help of medical science, ageing can be delayed and reversed to some extent. Rejuvenation is a medical discipline focused on the practical reversal of the ageing process. Skin rejuvenation can be achieved either surgically or non-surgically.

Methods available

Ablative lasers

The use of laser technologies dates back to the early 1960s for skin disorders. Soon they were utilized for aesthetic purposes. Ablative CO_2 was introduced around 1980 but the results were mixed due to many side effects.[1]

Later, pulsed and scanned CO_2 and Er:YAG was introduced, which were associated with fewer side effects. Ablative lasers are considered the most effective in skin rejuvenation but associated adverse effects are increased, due to epidermal damage. Long-term studies of histopathology after CO_2 and Er:YAG showed reorganization of collagen and elastin in the dermis, mainly with some changes in the epidermis.[2-6] On the basis of these results it was thought that non-ablative lasers can improve photoaging by dermal collagen remodelling and ablative lasers can help in skin resurfacing and collagen remodelling.

Ablative fractional lasers

In the first decade of the 2000s, laser development led to the introduction of ablative fractional lasers. Lasers per se are intelligent mechanical devices that identify their chromophore very specifically. Their mechanism of action is quite unique. They produce microthermal treatment zones (MTZ) in the epidermis and dermis depending on the type and settings of the laser. Areas adjacent to MTZ are normal, which helps in fast healing in fractional lasers.[7] Dermal penetration of the fractional laser leads to remodelling of collagen, as well as neocollagenesis by surrounding fibroblasts. In general, fractional lasers are better than conventional ablative ones because of shorter downtime, early recovery and fewer side effects.

Microneedling

Microneedling is percutaneous collagen induction therapy. Microneedling involves fine needles that cause micro-dermal wounds. These micro-injuries lead to the formation of new collagen, remodelling of existing collagen and neovascularization of papillary dermis which ultimately lead to a reduction of skin wrinkles and laxity.

Radiofrequency resurfacing

Radiofrequency (RF) resurfacing in rejuvenation can be invasive or non-invasive. It acts on the dermis without affecting the epidermis. Monopolar RF employs heat generation by electromagnetic energy within a target tissue. The heat production results in the skin tightening within the dermal tissue by denaturation and contraction of collagen fibres, and initiates new collagen formation in subsequent weeks.

Microneedling with radiofrequency is a minimally invasive procedure that delivers the energy through insulated or non-insulated microneedles to the dermis without much damage to the epidermis. It gives good results with minimum downtime, and fewer side effects.

Others

Topical retinol derivatives – these have been used for a long time for skin rejuvenation. They are also used as maintenance therapy after other procedural therapies for skin rejuvenation.

Chemical peels – peels act by creating controlled shedding of skin with the goal of stimulating the new skin growth through the growth of epidermal layers along with improvement of the texture. Glycolic acid, lactic acid, phenol, azelaic acid and retinol peels either alone or in combination with other modalities are the most commonly used peels. They address uneven skin tone, open pores, wrinkles and laxity.

Microdermabrasion – this is a simple procedure using aluminium oxide or other crystals. Crystals have an abrasive property that injures the stratum corneum. The healing process brings new cells, and the skin feels smoother. Microdermabrasion can be combined with other procedures.

Hydrafacials have been more popular of late, these work on principles of dermabrasion, electric stimulation and electroporation of meso solutions, restoring rejuvenation and hydration of the skin.

Table 1: Role of PRP in skin rejuvenation

Indications	**Mechanism of action**	**Method**	**Results**
Skin rejuvenation Rhytids Photodamaged skin Periorbital hyperpigmentation Breast augmentation Vulvovaginal rejuvenation	Increased proliferation of human dermal fibroblasts and stimulation of collagen synthesis Increased expression of matrix metalloproteinases (MMP) enhances the removal of photodamaged ECM Increases expression of G1 cell cycle regulators accelerates wound healing Accelerates hyaluronic acid production – improves skin hydration	A topical application under occlusion Direct intradermal injections As an adjuvant to lasers or microneedling	Improves skin quality, elasticity and firmness Significant improvement in fine wrinkles – nasolabial folds > crow's feet > transverse forehead lines Lower erythema index Reduces transient adverse effects and decrease the downtime associated with lasers Improves skin volume and turgor

How PRP works in skin rejuvenation

PRP is a rich source of growth factors and cytokines, stored in the α-granules of platelets including platelet-derived growth factors (PDGF), transforming growth factors (TGF), vascular endothelial growth factors (VEGF) and insulin-like growth factors (IGF) of platelets. PRP is also rich in several cell adhesion molecules such as fibrin, fibronectin and vitronectin, which are responsible for cell migration and provide a scaffolding for the tissues. PRP increases the expression of G1 cell cycle regulatory proteins, which accelerate wound healing. Matrix metalloproteinase (MMP) 1 and 3 help to remove the photodamaged extracellular matrix (ECM). A dose-response relationship has been identified in vitro between platelet concentration and human adult mesenchymal stem cell proliferation, fibroblast proliferation and type I collagen production.[8] PRP also helps in reducing pigmentation. According to a study conducted by Kim et al. on mice, TGF-β inhibits melanin synthesis.[9]

Kim et al. studied the effect of PRP on collagen production by fibroblasts. They found a remodelling of ECM, which is essential for skin rejuvenation. There was increased expression of collagen, MMP-1 and mRNA in fibroblasts.[10]

PRP monotherapy

PRP may be injected intradermally or sub-dermally to induce collagen production to enhance skin colour and texture, and decrease the appearance of fine lines. In general, treatment sessions are performed at four to six-week intervals for three to five months, or until the desired result is achieved.

In a six-month study at Benha University involving 20 females, three sessions of intradermal PRP injections were given. Results were evaluated by photographs, subjective assessment and the physician's impression. Results were good in terms of skin homogeneity. No serious side effects were noted.[11]

In a study by Redaelli et al., the effect of PRP on face and neck rejuvenation was conducted for three months with 23 patients. They were given injections of PRP at monthly intervals. After one month of the final session, the results were obtained and they found PRP very promising in rejuvenation.[12]

A study by Elnehrawy et al. on 20 volunteers with a single intradermal PRP injection showed that PRP was well tolerated and efficient in the rejuvenation of the skin. There was an improvement in wrinkles, especially around nasolabial folds.[13]

PRP can also be used for volume augmentation by injecting it into the deep dermis. By biostimulation, PRP provides natural-looking volumization of the face.[14]

Bio fillers utilizing platelet-poor plasma are cost-effective, temporary solutions for volumizing the face and are slowly gaining popularity.

PRP with other modalities

PRP with fractional lasers

Fractional CO_2 laser is being used for rejuvenation with good safety and effectiveness. It works on the principle of selective photothermolysis. Fractional CO_2 creates microthermal damaged zones with controllable depth, width and density. These microthermal damaged areas are like vertical wounds, and adding PRP to it helps in wound healing and early recovery of the treatment area due to the presence of its multiple growth factors. Moreover, PRP is associated with increased collagen expression and fibroblast proliferation, one of the main mechanisms of skin rejuvenation. A randomized controlled trial by Hui et al. studied the combined effect of fractional CO_2 with PRP versus fractional CO_2 alone on 13 females. All of them underwent fractional CO_2 laser, following which (randomly) half of the face was injected with PRP, and the other half was injected with normal saline. They found that combined application of fractional CO_2 and PRP effectively reduced the wrinkles and PRP also helped reduce the side effects of CO_2, such as erythema and pigmentation.[15]

In one Korean study, 25 subjects were used to see the effect of PRP after a fractional CO_2 laser on the inner arm. They all underwent CO_2 resurfacing followed by random application of PRP and normal saline. They concluded there was less erythema, and rapid healing following combined fractional CO_2 and PRP.[16]

Shin et al. studied the effect of PRP combined with fractional Er:YAG laser. Twenty-two females were enrolled in the study; half of them were treated with fractional Er:YAG laser and the rest were treated with fractional Er:YAG laser followed by topical application of PRP. This study showed that combination treatment with PRP and fractional laser resulted in objective improvement of skin elasticity, a lower erythema index and an increase in collagen density as well.[17]

Our experience

We use PRP therapy along with the Er:YAG laser. A combination of PRP and Er:YAG laser is used at monthly intervals for three months. It gives good and efficacious results in terms of reducing fine lines and overall improvement of skin texture. (Figure 1)

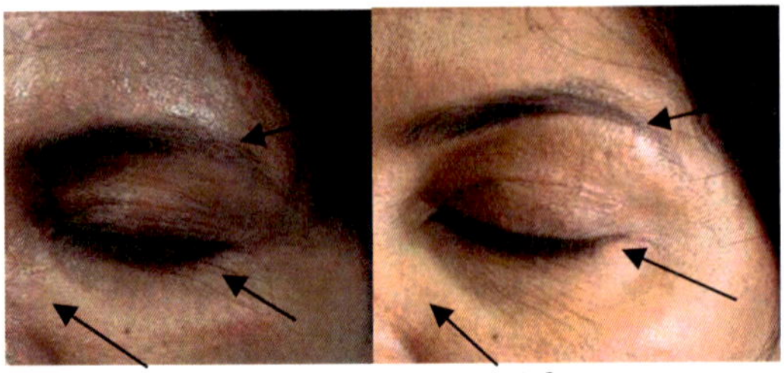

Figure 1: Results of combined therapy of Er:YAG laser and PRP at four-week intervals for three months. Improvement can be seen in skin texture, wrinkles and brow lift.

PRP with microneedling (Box 1)

Microneedling temporarily disrupts and bypasses the formidable bilayered lipid barrier of the stratum corneum. The production of numerous micro-channels in the dermis activates normal wound healing. Micropunctures are created using microneedles which produce a controlled skin injury without actually damaging the epidermis. These micro-injuries cause minimal superficial bleeding and trigger wound healing cascade with the release of various growth factors such as PDGF, TGF-α and TGF-β, connective tissue activating protein, connective tissue growth factor, and fibroblast growth factor (FGF). The use of PRP with microneedling can boost this process and reduce the recovery time.

Yuksel et al. used PRP with dermaroller and intradermal injection for skin rejuvenation on ten subjects. PRP was applied over the face after doing the dermaroller and injected intradermally into the crow's feet. They found it a safe and effective modality for rejuvenation.[18]

Box 1: Practical points for microneedling and PRP injections

---

1. Topical anaesthesia using topical numbing creams should be used to minimize pain.
    - Topical numbing should extend all the way to the edge of the hairline as well as to the edge of the tragus.
    - Numbing cream should be applied 45–60 minutes before the procedure, numbing can be done concurrently while waiting for the blood to be spun and processed.

2. Microneedling for various areas should be done at different depths because the skin of the face, neck and chest varies in its thickness.
   - Each individual, their skin texture and sebaceous quality should be taken into account, with patients with thicker skin able to have microneedling performed at greater depths.
     - Forehead: 1 to 1.5 mm
     - Periorbital: 0.5 to 1.5 mm
     - Face: 1.5 to greater than 2 mm
     - Nasal skin, especially over the upper dorsum: 0.5 to 1 mm
     - Neck and décolleté: 0.5 to 1.5 mm
   - As the needles oscillate, they will automatically puncture the skin to the desired depth, and additional pressure does not need to be used while using microneedling devices.
   - It is important to avoid additional pressure and dragging the device along the skin because that can cause deeper line injuries, irregularity and unevenness.
3. Microneedling with PRP and injections of PRP can be combined during the same treatment. For most patients, microneedling will help the overall skin texture, whereas injections will further help collagen stimulation from the deeper tissues.
4. Tips for reducing pain during the procedure:
   - Use of small needles such as a 32- or a 34-gauge needle will help with discomfort.
   - Slow injection is recommended during the procedure.
   - Ice-packs or vibration devices can improve patient comfort during the procedure.
5. Patients with a history of cold sores should take prophylaxis with an antiviral drug before the procedure to prevent a flare-up after microneedling and PRP injections.

Microneedling utilizes multiple fine needles which can penetrate up to the papillary and reticular dermis to mechanically induce angiogenesis, elastin and collagen production, resulting in wound healing and skin remodelling while preserving the epidermal barrier. PRP may be applied to the skin immediately after MN to improve skin texture and elasticity though injectable PRP gives better outcome in terms of lift and firmness. (Figure 2)

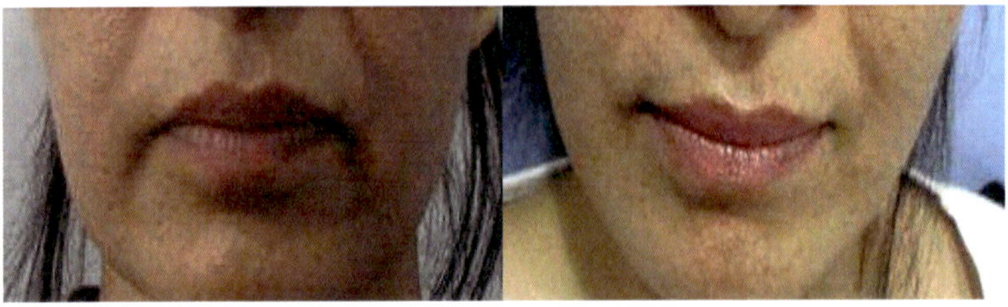

Before After

Figure 2: Improvement in nasolabial and mesomental folds after two sessions of MNRF and PRP therapy (Photo: Dr Suruchi Garg, Aura Skin Institute, Chandigarh)

Studies report good results with monthly PRP injections for three consecutive months for infraorbital rejuvenation. Improvement was noted in terms of patient satisfaction, infraorbital wrinkles, decrease in erythema and the melanin index.[19] Similar results have been observed in our experience. (Figure 3)

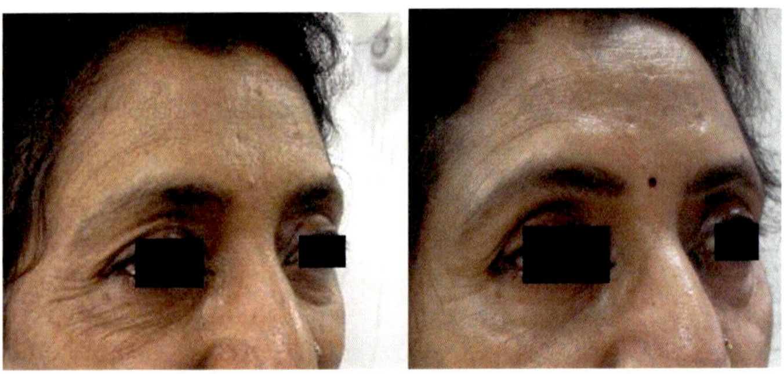

Before After

Figure 3: Periorbital rejuvenation after two sessions of MNRF and PRP therapy (Photo: Dr Suruchi Garg, Aura Skin Institute, Chandigarh)

By using MNRF in volume restoration mode by lifting and filling fat planes against the plane of their descent, overall age reversal of 10 years was attained based on the global drooping and wrinkle (DW) scoring system. (Photo: Dr Suruchi Garg, Aura Skin Institute, Chandigarh)

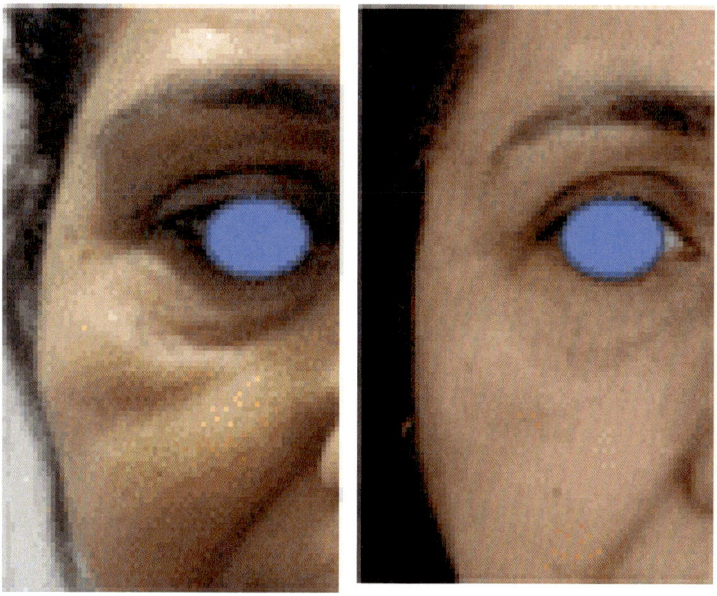

Figure 4: Periorbital rejuvenation after two sessions of MNRF and PRP therapy. There is improvement in volume deficit, the nasojugal groove and tear trough compartments. Based on global drooping and wrinkle classification, the periorbital area improved from grade 4 to grade 2, malar fat from grade 4 to grade 2 and temple area from grade 3 to grade 1, and nasolabial folds from grade 4 to grade 3.

PRP with hyaluronic acid

As mentioned previously, there is a significant decrease in hyaluronic acid level in aged skin, so hyaluronic acid can be used for rejuvenation. In a study of 94 females by Ulusal et al., the combination of PRP and hyaluronic acid injections improved facial skin with noticeable and statistically substantial enhancement. The improvements are more noteworthy with a higher number of injections.[20]

Conclusion

PPR has good evidence behind its use for skin rejuvenation, especially when combined with other treatment modalities, including microneedling or laser therapy.

PRP has been reported to improve dermal elasticity and skin texture via the stimulation of dermal fibroblast stimulation and the expression of matrix metalloproteinases (MMP) 1 and 3. Furthermore, it accelerates hyaluronic acid production and leads to improvement in skin hydration and volumization. Various methods have been employed for the application of PRP including intradermal or topical PRP alone, or in combination with microneedling with promising results.

References

1. Airan LE, Hruza G. Current lasers in skin resurfacing. *Facial Plast Surg Clin North Am.* 2005;**13**:127-139.
2. Kaufmann R, Hibst R. Pulsed erbium: YAG laser ablation in cutaneous surgery. *Lasers Surg Med.* 1996;**19**:324-330.
3. Kuo T, Speyer MT, Ries WR, Reinisch L. Collagen thermal damage and collagen synthesis after cutaneous laser resurfacing. *Lasers Surg Med.* 1998;**23**:66-71.
4. Kauvar AN, Geronemus RG. Histology of laser resurfacing. *Dermatol Clin.* 1997;**15**:459-467.
5. Alster TS, Kauvar AN, Geronemus RG. Histology of high-energy pulsed CO_2 laser resurfacing. *Semin Cutan Med Surg.* 1996;**15**:189-193.
6. Kauvar AN, Waldorf HA, Geronemus RG. A histopathological comparison of "charfree" carbon dioxide lasers. *Dermatol Surg.* 1996;**22**:343-348.
7. Alexiades-Armenakas MR, Dover JS, Arndt KA. Fractional laser skin resurfacing. *J Drugs Dermatol.* 2012;**11**:1274-1287.
8. Kakudo N, Minakata T, Mitsui T, Kushida S, Notodihardjo FZ, Kusumoto K. Proliferation-promoting effect of platelet-rich plasma on human adipose-derived stem cells and human dermal fibroblasts. *Plast Reconstr Surg.* 2008;**122**:1352–60.
9. Kim DS, Park SH, Park KC. Transforming growth factor-beta1 decreases melanin synthesis via delayed extracellular signal regulated kinase activation. *Int J Biochem Cell Biol* 2004;**36**:1482-1491.
10. Kim DH, Je YJ, Kim CD, Lee YH, Seo YJ, Lee JH, et al. Can platelet-rich plasma be used for skin rejuvenation? Evaluation of effects of platelet-rich plasma on human dermal fibroblast. *Ann Dermatol* 2011;**23**:424-431.
11. Mikhael NW, El-Esawy FM. Skin rejuvenation with autologous concentrated platelet-rich plasma. *Egypt J Dermatol Venerol* 2014;**34**:5-9

12. Redaelli A, Romano D, Marcianó A. Face and neck revitalization with platelet rich plasma: clinical outcome in a series of 23 consecutively treated patients. *J Drugs Dermatol*. 2010;**9**:466-472.
13. Elnehrawy NY, Ibrahim ZA, Eltoukhy AM, Nagy HM. Assessment of the efficacy and safety of single platelet-rich plasma injection on different types and grades of facial wrinkles. *J Cosmet Dermatol* 2017; **16**:103-111.
14. Zenker S. Platelet rich plasma (PRP) for facial rejuvenation. *J Mèd Esth et Chir Derm*. 2010;**37**:179-183.
15. Hui Q, Chang P, Guo B, Zhang Y, Tao K. The clinical efficacy of autologous platelet-rich plasma combined with ultra-pulsed fractional CO_2 laser therapy for facial rejuvenation. *Rejuvenation Res*. 2017;**20**:25-31. doi:10.1089/rej.2016.1823.
16. Na J-I, Choi J-W, Choi H-R, Jeong J-B, Park K-C, Youn S-W, et al. Rapid healing and reduced erythema after ablative fractional carbon dioxide laser resurfacing combined with the application of autologous platelet-rich plasma. *Dermatol Surg*. 2011;**37**:463-8.
17. Min-Kyung S, Jong-Ho L, Sang-Jun L, Nack-In K. Platelet-rich plasma combined with fractional laser therapy for skin rejuvenation. *Dermatol Surg* 2012;**38**:623-630.
18. Yuksel EP, Sahin G, Aydin F, Senturk N, Turanli AY. Evaluation of effects of platelet-rich plasma on human facial skin. *J Cosmet Laser Ther* 2014;**16**:206-208.
19. Marx RE. Platelet-rich plasma (PRP): what is PRP and what is not PRP? *Implant Dent*. 2001;**10**:225-8.
20. Ulusal BG. Platelet-rich plasma and hyaluronic acid—An efficient biostimulation method for face rejuvenation. *J Cosmet Dermatol* 2017; **16**:112-119.

CHAPTER 11

THE ROLE OF PLATELET-RICH PLASMA (PRP) IN DISORDERS OF PIGMENTATION

ANKITA TUKNAYAT, DEVI MENON,
ANUVA BANSAL, SURUCHI GARG

Introduction

Facial hyperpigmentation, a common presentation of Indian patients, apart from being a cosmetic concern is also a challenge for the treating physicians. A wide variety of treatment options are available including topical agents, chemical peels, lasers, systemic drugs such as tranexamic acid, and other natural therapies. Although effective in most cases, some of these modalities are associated with adverse effects, and patient satisfaction also tends to vary with the various therapies.[1] Newer treatment options and techniques have become available over the past few years to overcome these limitations.

Platelet-rich plasma (PRP), which is a combination of multiple fundamental growth factors (GFs) and plasma proteins, is one such promising and safe therapy that could help pave the way for newer treatment options.[2]

Disorders of facial hyperpigmentation

There are numerous causes of hyperpigmentation. The common ones are as follows.

Melasma

Melasma is a common acquired pigmentary skin disorder characterized by symmetrical hyperpigmented macules. The exact cause of melasma is not yet known but the established pathogenetic factors implicated include genetics, sunlight, cosmetics, pregnancy, hormonal treatments, thyroid dysfunction and drugs.[3] In a more recent article by Garg et al., it was observed that almost all the patients with pigmentary disorders such as melasma have a dietary history of low protein intake. The authors were of the opinion that poor amino acid supply limits the capacity of the skin to repair the photodamage and decreases the keratinocyte turnover rate along with the accumulation of melanin.[4] (Figure 1)

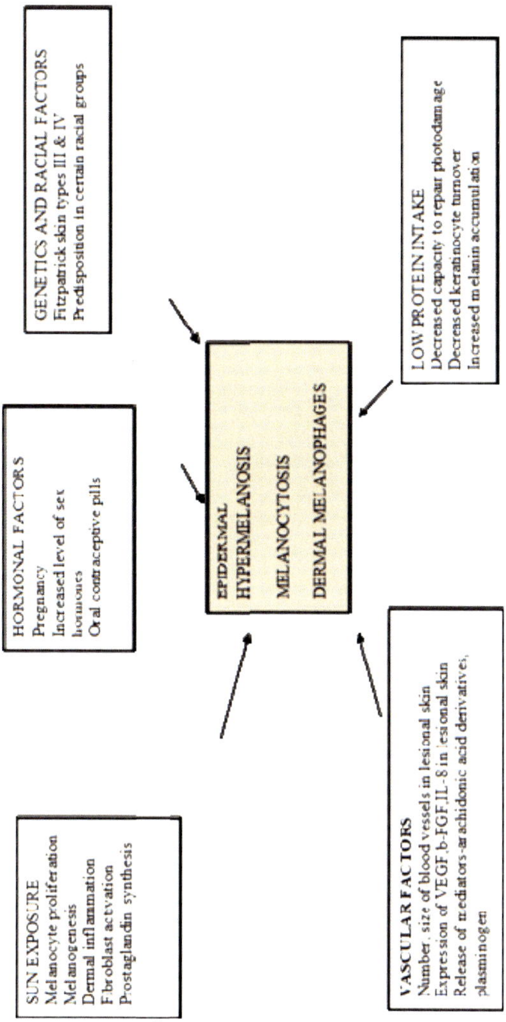

Figure 1-Aetiology of melasma[5]

Lichen planus pigmentosus (LPP)

LPP is characterized by generally asymptomatic, diffuse hyper pigmented patches present mostly over exposed areas and flexures. The exact aetiology is not known, although sunlight, cosmetics, hair dyes, mustard oil and hepatitis C have been implicated. Few topical and systemic treatment modalities are available; however, the pigmentation is generally recalcitrant to conventional therapy.[6]

Periorbital melanosis (POM)

This is characterized by variegated brown to almost black discoloration around the eyes.[4] The aetiological factors responsible for POM include dermal melanin deposition, post-inflammatory hyperpigmentation (atopic/allergic contact dermatitis), shadowing from lax skin and infraorbital swelling. A protein-poor diet also leads to decreased collagen turnover resulting in increased periorbital skin laxity and capillary fragility, which may trigger the vascular component of POM and aggravate the melanocytic pigmentation.

Post-inflammatory hyperpigmentation (PIH)

PIH is the most common pigmentary disorder in patients with skin type IV–VI. The lesions occur at the site of a previous inflammatory insult therefore the body surface area involved can be significant, particularly in patients with widespread diseases. Most lesions are a combination of epidermal and dermal pigment deposition. Without treatment, epidermal pigmentation can take months or years to resolve, and dermal pigmentation takes years to fade.[7]

Erythema dyschromium perstans (EDP)

EDP is an idiopathic, acquired and chronic skin disorder characterized by numerous asymptomatic, persistent hyperpigmented patches on the trunk, face and extremities, which can affect any age group. The aetiology of EDP is unknown. The pigmentation in EDP is due to the presence of melanin in the melanosome complexes in the dermis and in the epidermis. A variety of possible causative agents have been reported including ingestion of ammonium nitrate, orally administered X-ray contrast media, exposure to chlorothalonil, chronic hepatitis C infection and exposure to environmental contaminants.

Current treatment options

First, the underlying cause of the disease should be identified, and corrective measures should be taken. It is also equally important to counsel the patients adequately about disease chronicity and the risk of recurrence. Currently available treatment options based on the standard guidelines are as follows[8]:

First-line treatment

These involve broad-spectrum sunscreen in combination with topical agents such as keratinocyte turnover stimulator (retinoids), tyrosinase inhibitor (hydroquinone, azelaic acid, arbutin), melanosome transfer inhibitor (retinoids, soybean trypsin inhibitor), and chelation of copper (kojic acid, ascorbic acid).[9]

Second-line treatment

These are chemical peels such as glycolic acid 20–70%, salicylic acid 20–30%, trichloroacetic acid (TCA) 10–25% and Jessner's solution.)

Third-line treatment

Lasers: the 1064 nm Q-switched, neodymium-doped yttrium aluminium garnet (Nd:YAG), and the 1550 nm Erbium-doped fibre fractional thermolysis lasers are those most frequently used.[10] Common treatments are mesotherapy, and microneedling radiofrequency (MNRF) plus mesotherapy.

Platelet-rich plasma (PRP) in the treatment of hyperpigmentation

Mechanism of action of PRP

Platelet-rich plasma (PRP) is a high concentration of platelets in a small volume of plasma. PRP contains various growth factors and cytokines released by platelets, and these substances play a critical role in all aspects of the wound healing process.[11] The most important contents of platelets are contained in the α-granules; there are more than 30 bioactive substances in these granules. Some of the bioactive substances present in the α-granules include platelet-derived growth factor (PDGF), transforming growth factor (TGF)-β1 and β2, epidermal growth factor (EGF), fibroblast growth factor (FGF) and vascular endothelial growth factor (VEGF)[12,13] (Figure 2).

Kim et al. investigated the effects of TGF-β1 on melanogenesis by using a spontaneously immortalized mouse melanocyte cell line. They found that TGF-β1 inhibits melanin synthesis via delayed extracellular signal-regulated kinase activation, which in turn reduces the activity of tyrosinase. TGFβ released upon PRP activation also stimulates basement membrane healing by laminin, collagen IV and tenascin, resulting in a pigment lightening effect.[14]

Yun et al. studied the effect of EGF on melanogenesis by using mouse-derived immortalized melanocytes from a laser-treated keratinocyte-conditioned culture media. They reported that normal human melanocytes and melan-A cells had substantial EGF receptor expression, and these receptors mediated the action of EGF to reduce inflammation-induced melanogenesis and hyperpigmentation.[15] The pigmentary improvement that occurs with PRP treatment may be associated with the increase in skin volume. PDGF has a significant role in blood vessel formation, and in the synthesis of collagen and components of the extracellular matrix, including hyaluronic acid. Hyaluronic acid has been shown to increase skin tone and volume, resulting in brighter skin.[16]

Thus, PRP has a multiple action as depicted in Figure 2.

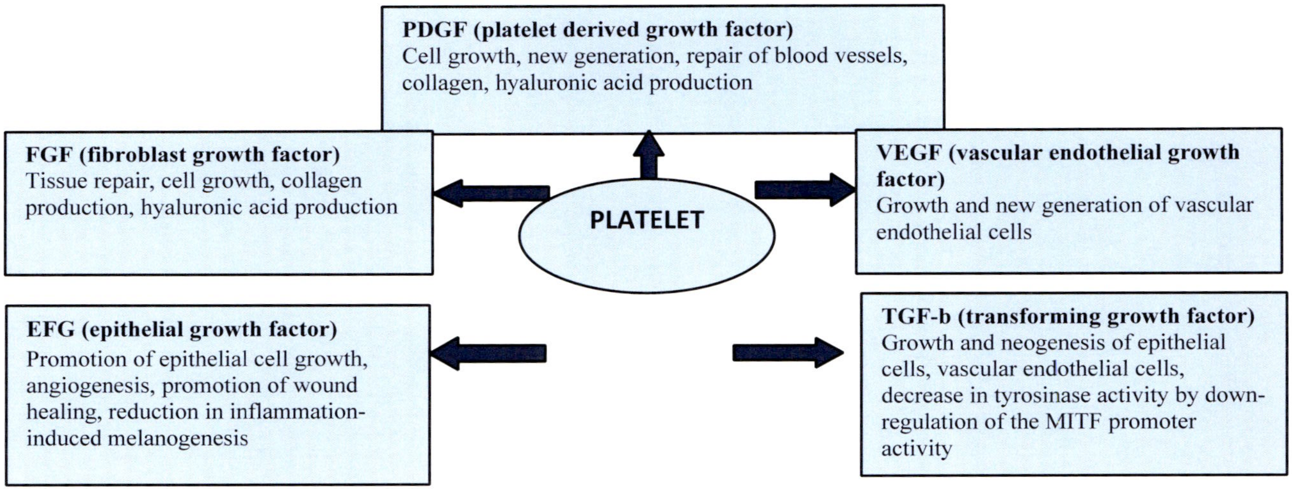

Figure 2: Growth factors in platelet-rich plasma responsible for reducing pigmentation

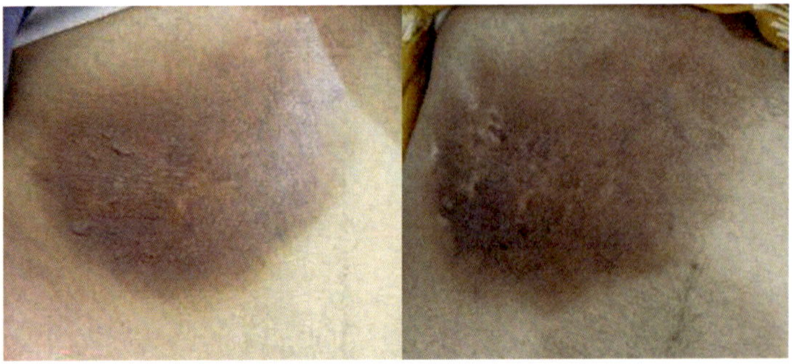

Figure 3: Plaque morphea over the abdomen, pre- and post-treatment with topical calcipotriol-steroid combination and five sessions of injectable PRP therapy, and Er:YAG laser over a period of a year. Although pigmentation has not improved much, there is a remarkable improvement in the itching, induration, texture of plaque, sensation of tightness, surrounding active violaceous border and the appearance of islands of normal skin.

Discussion

Though pigmentary disorders do not cause morbidity to the patient, they can be a significant cosmetic concern and can affect an individual's quality of life. The available therapeutic modalities, even if effective in most cases, come with a list of side effects and are not always satisfactory. PRP has emerged as a new treatment modality for several dermatological and aesthetic problems including alopecia, wound healing, skin rejuvenation, acne scars, striae distensae. Many studies also report the potential effect of PRP in the treatment of hyperpigmentation. Being an autologous preparation, PRP is devoid of any serious adverse effects, apart from local injection site reactions such as pain or secondary infection, which can be avoided with proper precautions, and the risk of transmission of infections such as hepatitis B, C or HIV has also not been observed.[17,18]

Various studies have been conducted to demonstrate the efficacy of PRP in pigmentary disorders. Eman et al. evaluated the value of PRP in the treatment of melasma in 23 adult patients using two different delivery techniques: microneedling using a dermapen versus microinjections using meso needles. They found a significant improvement in the Melasma Area and Severity Index (MASI) score following PRP treatment, but no significant difference in the two delivery modalities.[19]

A pilot study on 25 Korean subjects by Jung Na et al. demonstrated an improvement in the melanin index (the melanin index indicates the darkness of skin and is computed from the absorbed and reflected light intensities of red and infrared light) of patients treated with PRP in combination with ablative fractional photothermolysis.[11]

Ch et al. examined the effects of PRP in the treatment of melasma in conjunction with Q-switched Nd:YAG (1064 nm) and topical alpha-arbutin, administered at a monthly interval for two sessions in two cases of melasma. They reported about 33.5% and 20% improvement in the MASI scores of cases 1 and 2, respectively. The authors attributed the lower percentage of improvement in case 2 to the higher Fitzpatrick skin phototype (V) and the more resistant mixed type of melasma.[20]

In another study by Tsiatoura et al. on PRP and fractional CO_2 laser combination treatment for face rejuvenation at monthly interval for four sessions, 60% of the volunteers were found to have a reduction of irregular pigmentation.[21]

Mehryan et al. performed a study on 10 patients where a single session with intradermal injections of 1.5 ml platelet-rich plasma was given into the tear trough area and wrinkles of crow's feet. The effect was compared three months after treatment with baseline. They reported a statistically significant improvement in infraorbital colour homogeneity.[22, 23]

Garg et al. observed that when PRP was added to the topical regimen in a patient with melasma who was previously resistant to first- and second-line treatment modalities, there was a significant improvement in her MASI score.[24]

We believe that PRP has the following advantages, making it a promising treatment option for pigmentary disorders:

- It has an additive anti-ageing and skin remodelling effect as it promotes neocollagenesis and provides an environment for vascularization, which leads to higher patient satisfaction.
- PRP helps in decreasing the downtime, improves the hydration and incidence of adverse effects such as post-inflammatory hyperpigmentation, which may be associated with dry and desiccated skin with the usage of ablative lasers alone.
- Higher fluencies of lasers can be used.
- The result lasts longer, and after the intensive three sessions are over, maintenance sessions need to be repeated only once in six months to a year.
- If lasers or MNRF are being planned as monotherapy for the treatment of melasma, then a cocktail with PRP therapy may reduce the need for multiple sessions.

Our experience

At Aura skin institute, we initially assess the patients who present with complaints of pigmentation for any signs of dietary protein deficiency based on daily activities and physical workout, and advise corrective measures for the same, as we believe that protein is an essential macronutrient for optimal functioning and repair of the skin. Patients are advised to avoid prolonged starvation and especially avoid missing their breakfast. Patients already on intermittent fasting should not observe it beyond six months as there may be depletion of various micronutrients. We also suggest basic investigations such as thyroid function tests, vitamin D and B12 levels, iron studies and lipid profile, to rule out other nutritional deficiencies and dietary irregularities.

Global drooping and wrinkles scores[25] are calculated to assess the facial age and those having a score of less than 26 usually have surface changes so they are offered less aggressive therapies such as PRP with superficial MNRF (needle length less than 2 mm) or Er:YAG Pixel™ laser or Alma Hybrid laser (1570 nm) with impact infusion of PRP, thereby increasing the penetration and inducing mild inflammatory reactions. Those who have a score of >26 are given a cocktail treatment of peels, PRP, deep MNRF (needle depth more than 2 mm) and Alma Hybrid® (CO_2 and 1570 nm) with an impact infusion of PRP therapy for better results. During the post-procedure period, patients are kept on an early morning high protein diet (1–1.5 gm/kg body weight) rich in vitamins and minerals. They are given instructions to apply retinol and vitamin C-based topical applications and follow strict photoprotection. They are also advised not to use any chemical hair dyes and salon procedures during the treatment period.

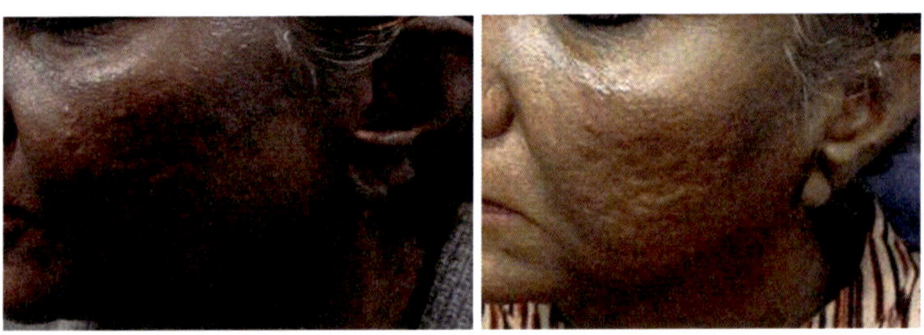

Figure 4: Pre- and post-procedure photographs of a patient with stable LPP treated with a cocktail of three sessions of Alma Er:YAG Pixel laser and injectable PRP repeated at four-week intervals.

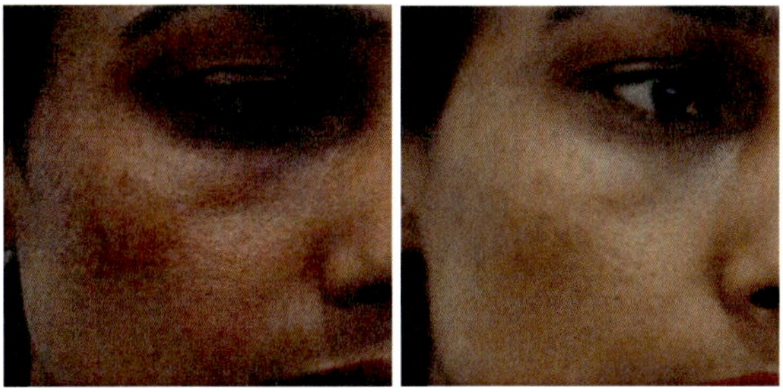

Figure 5: Pre- and post-procedure photographs of a patient with periorbital pigmentation and Malar melasma treated with a cocktail of three sittings of 50% glycolic acid (GA) peel, MNRF (de-age) plus PRP repeated at four-week intervals. There is also visible improvement in the periorbital ageing scale as per global drooping and wrinkle classification.[25] Periorbital hollowness improved from grade 3 to 2, and wrinkles from grade 3 to 2.

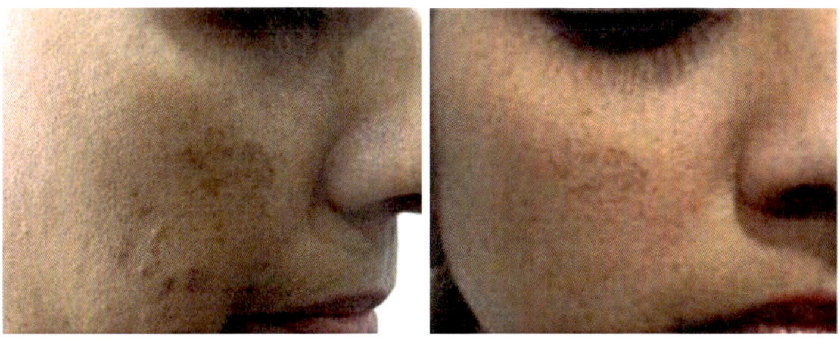

Figure 6: Pre- and post-procedural photographs of a patient with malar melasma treated with a cocktail of two sessions of PRP and Alma Pixel Q-switched Nd:YAG laser at four-week intervals.

Conclusion

Our personal experiences as well as existing literature on PRP in pigmentation lead us to believe that PRP is an invaluable adjuvant treatment option and should be considered an effective therapy for difficult-to-treat pigment disorders.

References

1. Khanna N, Rasool S. Facial melanoses: Indian perspective. *Indian J Dermatol Venereol Leprol.* 2011;**77**:552-64.
2. Bohara R, Bhamre N, Kshersagar J, Tardalkar K, Desai S, Despande M, et al. Platelet rich plasma: a potential treatment option in hyper pigmentation of skin. *Clin Surg.* 2018;**3**:1938.
3. Sarkar R, Gokhale N, Godse K, Ailawadi P, Arya L, Sarma N, et al. Medical management of melasma: a review with consensus recommendations by Indian pigmentary expert group. *Indian J Dermatol.* 2017;**62**:558-77 .
4. Garg S, Sangwan A. Dietary protein deficit and deregulated autophagy: a new clinico-diagnostic perspective in pathogenesis of early aging, skin, and hair disorders. *Indian Dermatol Online J* 2019;**10**:115-24.
5. Sonthalia S, Sarkar R. Etiopathogenesis of melasma. *Pigment Int.* 2015;*2*:21-7.
6. Khanna N, Rasool S. Facial melanoses: Indian perspective. *Indian J Dermatol Venereol Leprol.* 2011;**77**:552-64
7. Patel AB. Postinflammatory hyperpigmentation: review of pathogenesis, prevention, and treatment. *Pigment Int* 2014;**1**:59-69.
8. Desai SR. Hyperpigmentation therapy: a review. *J Clin Aesthet Dermatol*. 2014;**7**:13-7.
9. Chan R, Park KC, Lee MH, Lee ES. *Br J Dermatol*. 2008;**159**:697-703.
10. Kauvar AN. Successful treatment of melasma using a combination of microdermabrasion and Q-switched Nd:YAG lasers. *Lasers Surg Med.* 2012;**44**:117-124.
11. Na J-I, Choi J-W, Choi H-R, Jeong J-B, Park K-C, Youn S-W, et al. Rapid healing and reduced erythema after ablative fractional carbon dioxide laser resurfacing combined with the application of autologous platelet-rich plasma. *Dermatologic Surgery*. 2011;37:463-468.
12. Cayırlı M, Calışkan E, Açıkgöz G, Erbil AH, Ertürk G. Regression of melasma with platelet-rich plasma treatment. *Ann Dermatol.* 2014;**26**:401-2.
13. Bohara R, Bhamre N, Kshersagar J, Tardalkar K, Desai S, Despande M, et al. Platelet rich plasma: a potential treatment option in hyper pigmentation of skin. *Clin Surg*. 2018;**3**:1938.
14. Kim DS, Park SH, Park KC. Transforming growth factor-beta1 decreases melanin synthesis via delayed extracellular signal-regulated kinase activation. *Int J Biochem Cell Biol*. 2004;**36**:1482-1491.

15. Yun WJ, Bang SH, Min KH, Kim SW, Lee MW, Chang SE. Epidermal growth factor and epidermal growth factor signalling attenuate laser-induced melanogenesis. *Dermatol Surg.* 2013;**39**:1903-1911.
16. Papakonstantinou E, Roth M, Karakiulakis G. Hyaluronic acid: a key molecule in skin aging. *Dermatoendocrinol.* 2012;**4**:253-25.
17. Smiell JM, Wieman TJ, Steed DL, Perry BH, Sampson AR, Schwab BH. Efficacy and safety of becaplermin (recombinant human platelet-derived growth factor-BB) in patients with nonhealing, lower-extremity diabetic ulcers: a combined analysis of four randomized studies. *Wound Repair Regen.* 1999;**7**:335-46.
18. Al-Shami SH. Treatment of periorbital hyperpigmentation using platelet-rich plasma injections. *Am. J. Dermatol Venereol.* 2014;**3**:87-94.
19. Hofny ERM, Abdel-Motaleb AA, Ghazally A, Ahmed AM, Hussein MRA. Platelet rich plasma is a useful therapeutic option in melasma. *J Dermatolog Treat.* 2018;**30**:396-401.
20. Ch Y, Ramasamy TS, Amini F. Response to intradermal autologous platelet rich plasma injection in refractory dermal melasma: report of two cases. *Journal of Health and Translational Medicine (JUMMEC).* 2015;18:1-6.
21. Tsiatoura A, Vekris A, Zafeiratou D. Platelet-rich plasma and fractional CO_2 laser combination treatment for face rejuvenation. (2014). *J Am Acad Dermatol.* 2014;70: AB19.
22. Mehryan P, Zartab H, Rajabi A, Pazhoohi N, Firooz A. Assessment of efficacy of platelet-rich plasma (PRP) on infraorbital dark circles and crow's feet wrinkles. *J Cosmet Dermatol.* 2014;**13**:72-78.
23. Sarkar R, Ranjan R, Garg S, Garg VK, Sonthalia S, Bansal S. Periorbital hyperpigmentation: a comprehensive review. *J Clin Aesthet Dermatol.* 2016;**9**:49-55.
24. Garg S, Khillan K, Bharija SC. Platelet-rich plasma therapy in the treatment of recalcitrant melasma. *Dermatol Surg.* 2018;45:482-4.
25. Garg S, Khan N, Makadia S. Proposed global drooping and wrinkles classification and scoring system for aging face with validation and experience on 54 Indian subjects. *Indian J Dermatol Venereol Leprol.* 2018;**84**:672-7

CHAPTER 12

THE ROLE OF PLATELET-RICH PLASMA IN NON-HEALING ULCERS AND WOUNDS

CAROL LOBO, ANUVA BANSAL, SURUCHI GARG

Introduction

Chronic non-healing wounds are wounds that have failed to progress through the normal sequence of wound healing or proceed through the repair process without anatomic and functional restoration.[1] Non-healing ulcers and wounds are a major challenge to the healthcare system and cause significant morbidity. A comprehensive approach to wound care comprises overcoming factors that contribute to delayed healing. Platelet-rich plasma (PRP) is a cost-effective procedure and a breakthrough in the treatment of non-healing ulcers.

Wound healing

Wound healing is a dynamic and efficiently orchestrated process involved in the restoration of tissue integrity. It is divided into four phases: haemostasis, inflammatory phase, proliferative phase and remodelling. Following injury, the platelet clot formation and platelet degranulation with subsequent release of growth factors initiate the process of wound healing.[2]

Neutrophil chemotaxis followed by infiltration by macrophages at the wound site triggers the inflammatory process during the first two days of wound healing. In turn, activated macrophages and alpha granules of activated platelets release multiple growth factors, including platelet-derived growth factor (PDGF), transforming growth factors (TGF), interleukin-1 (IL-1) and fibroblast growth factor (FGF). Angiogenesis and fibroblastic activity are followed by collagen synthesis.[2,3] This process leads to an early increase in wound tensile strength, which is the most important parameter for healing of wounds, followed by epithelization and the ultimate remodelling process.

The phases of wound healing are controlled and regulated by growth factors, which exert a powerful influence on wound healing and repair. The growth factors involved in each phase of wound healing are depicted in Figure 1.

Factors affecting wound healing

Multiple intrinsic and extrinsic factors influence wound healing. Extrinsic factors such as infection, medications and venous stasis interfere with the wound healing process whereas intrinsic factors such as age, stress, diabetes, obesity, medications, alcoholism, smoking and nutrition affect the innate ability of the body to aid in adequate tissue repair. Factors affecting wound healing are listed in Table 1.

Figure 1 (next page): Phases of wound healing and growth factors involved
*PDGF: platelet-derived growth factor; TGF-β: transforming growth factor-beta; G-CSF: granulocyte – colony-stimulating factor; FGF: fibroblast growth factor; VEGF: vascular endothelial growth factor; EGF: epidermal growth factor; IGF: insulin-like growth factor.

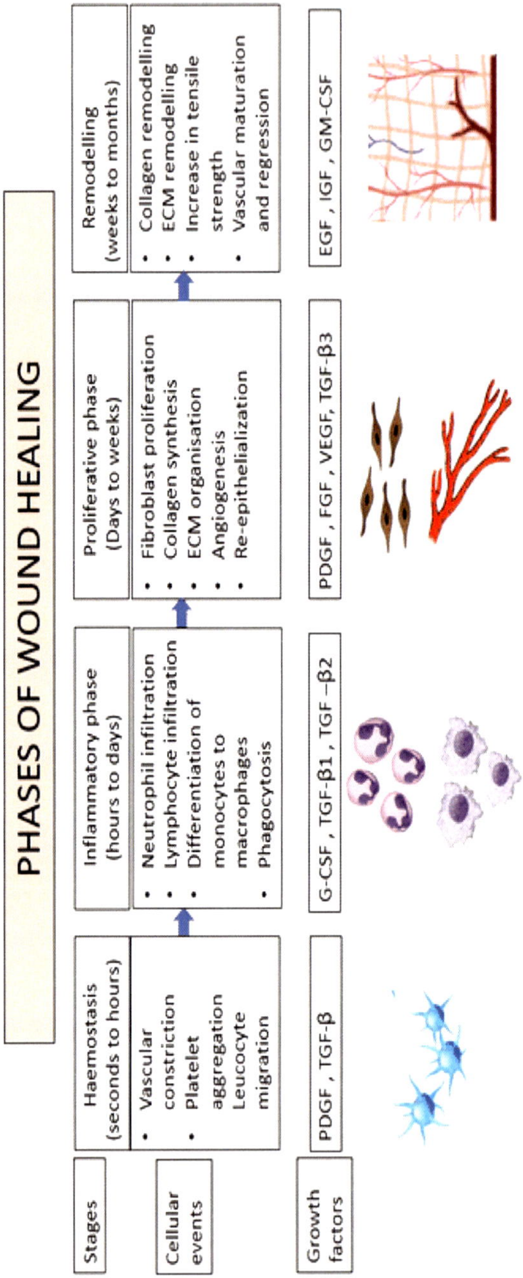
PHASES OF WOUND HEALING
Stages
Cellular events
Growth factors
Haemostasis (seconds to hours)
• Vascular constriction
• Platelet aggregation Leucocyte migration
PDGF , TGF-β
Inflammatory phase (hours to days)
• Neutrophil infiltration
• Lymphocyte infiltration
• Differentiation of monocytes to macrophages
• Phagocytosis
G-CSF , TGF-β1 , TGF –β2
Proliferative phase (Days to weeks)
• Fibroblast proliferation
• Collagen synthesis
• ECM organisation
• Angiogenesis
• Re-epithelialization
PDGF , FGF , VEGF, TGF-β3
Remodelling (weeks to months)
• Collagen remodelling
• ECM remodelling
• Increase in tensile strength
• Vascular maturation and regression
EGF , IGF , GM-CSF

Table 1: Factors affecting wound healing

INTRINSIC FACTORS	EXTRINSIC FACTORS
• advanced age • stress • malnutrition • vitamin deficiencies: vitamins A,C • mineral deficiencies: zinc, iron • diseases: atherosclerosis, cardiac or renal failure • alcoholism, smoking • immunocompromised states: cancer, diabetes mellitus, HIV/AIDS	• local infection • ischaemia: circulation, local tension • medications: glucocorticoids, chemotherapeutic drugs, NSAIDs, ionizing radiation • venous insufficiency

*HIV/AIDS: Human immunodeficiency virus/acquired immunodeficiency syndrome; NSAIDS: non-steroidal anti-inflammatory drugs

Chronic ulcers and non-healing ulcers

Chronic ulcers or non-healing ulcers are defined as spontaneous or traumatic lesions, typically in the lower extremities, which are either unresponsive to initial therapy or persist despite appropriate care and do not proceed towards healing in a defined period of time with an underlying aetiology that may be related to systemic disease or local disorders.[4] A range of four weeks to three months has been used to define chronic wounds in the literature.[5]

The Wound Healing Society classifies chronic wounds into four major categories[6]:

1. pressure ulcers
2. diabetic foot ulcers
3. venous ulcers
4. arterial insufficiency ulcers

Chronic wounds are characterized by a prolonged inflammatory phase and aberrant growth factor activities, leading to failure of normal wound healing with the potential for infections. Recurrent secondary infections,[7] drug-resistant microbial biofilms[8] and the inability of dermal and epidermal cells to respond to reparative stimuli for healing are common to all the above non-healing ulcers.[9]

Molecular basis of non-healing ulcers

Secondary wound infections result in a pro-inflammatory micro-environment, particularly high concentrations of inflammatory infiltrate and increased protease activity. In addition, local tissue hypoxia and repeated wound infections promote higher levels of matrix metalloproteases (MMP) 2, 8 and 9, resulting in decreased growth factor functions and levels, and decreased levels of tissue inhibitor MMP 1. This leads to prolonged inflammation and increased collagenolytic activity.[10,11] The combination of increased pro-inflammatory cytokines and an abnormally prolonged inflammatory phase culminates in wound chronicity.

A chronically inflamed wound micro-environment degrades and sequesters proteins and cytokines, especially growth factors such as PDGF, EGF and TGF-β.[2] Cooper et al. demonstrated a marked reduction of growth factors in chronic wounds compared to acute wounds.[5] Decreased growth factor levels and upregulation of pro-inflammatory cytokines and chemokines hinder the normal progression of wound healing and consequently the potential for full wound closure. The micro-environment in chronic wounds must thus be modified to eliminate the factors impeding healing as well as to provide an effective intervention towards wound healing. A dual approach targeting correction of any underlying systemic disease and wound-micro-environmental tissue therapy is vital.

Reasons for using PRP

Platelet-rich plasma (PRP) is a first-generation plasma concentrate containing 95% platelets, 4% red blood cells and 1% white blood cells. Ehrenfest et al. classified PRP into four main types[12]:

1. Pure platelet-rich plasma (P-PRP): a preparation rich in platelets and devoid of leukocytes and low-density fibrin network after activation;
2. Leukocyte and platelet-rich plasma (L-PRP): a preparation rich in platelets and leukocytes, and with a low-density fibrin network;
3. Pure platelet-rich fibrin (P-PRF) or leukocyte-poor platelet-rich fibrin: a preparation containing high-density fibrin network and without leucocytes;
4. Leukocyte and platelet-rich fibrin (L-PRF): a preparation containing leukocytes and with a high-density fibrin network.

Upon activation of PRP, the degranulation of alpha granules present within the platelets releases growth factors and cytokines. Growth factors attract stem cells and attach to specific tyrosine kinase receptors on the cell membrane, leading to activation of secondary messenger proteins through signalling cascade, which then enter the cell nucleus and influence the expression of the genes responsible for triggering mitosis, angiogenesis and macrophage activation.[13] The reasons for using PRP in non-healing ulcers is the delivery of concentrated platelet-derived growth factors to accelerate the wound healing process. These growth factors include platelet-derived growth factor (PDGF), epidermal growth factor (EGF), fibroblast growth factor (FGF), insulin-like growth factor (IGF-1, IGF2) and vascular endothelial growth factor (VEGF) as shown in Figure 2.[14] Transforming growth factor-beta (TGFβ) promotes matrix and collagen synthesis. Platelet-derived growth factor (PDGF) is a chemoattractant and promotes cell proliferation and differentiation. Insulin growth factor-I (IGF-I) promotes cell proliferation and soft tissue growth. Fibroblast growth factor (FGF) induces angiogenesis and fibroblast proliferation. Endothelial growth factor (EGF) promotes cell proliferation, and vascular endothelial growth factor (VEGF) promotes angiogenesis.[2]

In addition, the fibrin network generated following platelet activation contributes to tissue repair, by providing a scaffold to the cells participating in the wound healing process at the site of injury.

The advantage of PRP is that it stimulates and accelerates the soft tissue healing, thereby creating a conducive environment for the restoration of affected tissue.[4]

Figure 2: Growth factors in PRP countering challenges in non-healing wounds

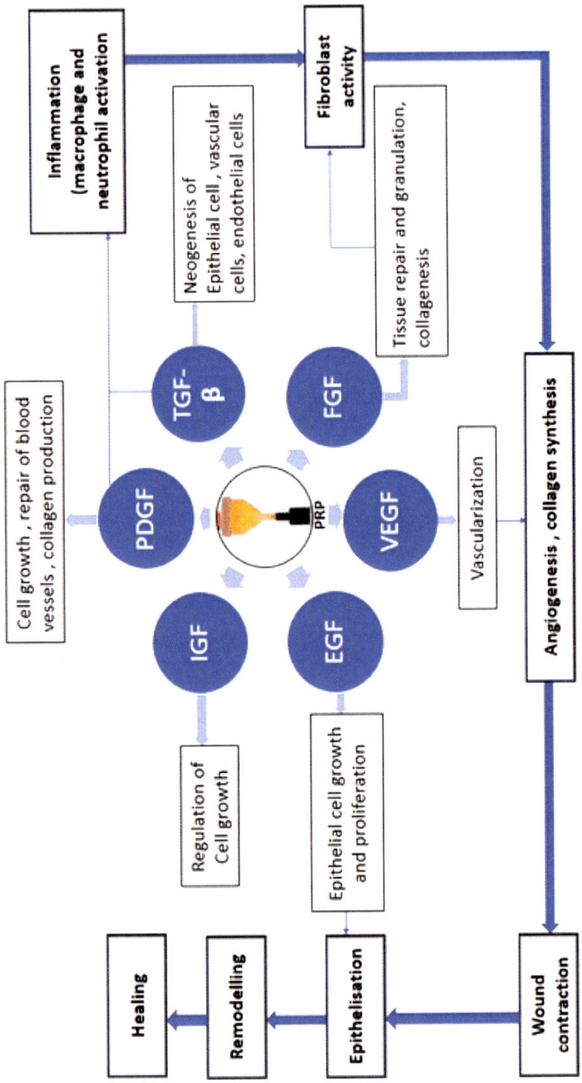

*PDGF: platelet-derived growth factor; TGF-β: transforming growth factor-beta; G-CSF: granulocyte colony-stimulating factor; FGF: fibroblast growth factor; VEGF: vascular endothelial growth factor; EGF: epidermal growth factor; IGF: insulin-like growth factor.

Studies and review of literature of PRP in wound healing

Knighton et al.[15] demonstrated the first clinical application of platelet-derived preparations in chronic leg ulcers. Following this, several platelet preparations have been used in solution, gel or by injection in wounds of varying aetiologies.[4,13,16–18]

A meta-analysis by Hu et al.[19] included eight RCTs involving 431 participants with chronic ulcers. Compared with controls, PRP was associated with a significantly increased ratio of complete ulcer healing and reduced areas of ulcers without significant adverse effects.

Another study in 56 patients with diabetic foot ulcers demonstrated a cure rate of 86% in the group treated with PRP (n=28) compared to 68% in the group treated with conventional topical antibiotic alone (n=28).[20]

Mohammadi et al. conducted a prospective cohort study of 70 diabetic patients with chronic diabetic foot ulcers. Topical activated autologous PRP gel applied weekly for four weeks significantly decreased the mean ulcer area to 51.9% of baseline (P=.008).[21]

Kakagia et al.[22] found a statistically higher rate of healing in chronic diabetic foot ulcers of 51 patients for the combination of PRP and protease-modulating matrix compared to protease-modulating matrix alone ($p<0.05$).

In another study,[18] activated PRP was sprayed on chronic ulcers until either complete healing took place or up to a maximum of six sittings, whichever occurred first; 46 patients (92%) showed complete healing. The mean time for ulcer healing was 4.38 weeks.

In a recent meta-analysis supporting the use of PRP in ulcer healing, 17 randomized controlled trials (RCTs) were included. PRP significantly increased the fraction and percentage of healed ulcers compared with the control group. In terms of the safety profile, the autologous PRP subgroup had a statistically significant and better safety profile compared to the homologous PRP subgroup.[23] Various studies demonstrating the efficacy of PRP in non-healing ulcers are shown in Table 2.

Table 2: Summary of studies using PRP in treatment of chronic wounds

Study	Study design	Type of ulcers	Number of pts	Treatment duration	Frequency of application	Result
Kakagia et al[22]	Randomised controlled trial	Diabetic foot ulcers >= 2.5 cm in any one dimension	51 Group A:ORC* Group B:PRP Group C: PRP+CRC*	8 weeks	Once/week	Significantly greater reduction of all three dimensions of the ulcers in Group C compared to other two groups (P<.001)
Jeong et al[24]	Prospective study	Chronic diabetic foot ulcers	100	2 weeks	Twice/week	Complete wound healing in 79 % pts from PRP treated group vs 46 % in the control group [p < 0.05). Time to complete wound healing was significantly lesser in the PRP group
Kontopodis et al[25]	Retrospective study	Chronic wounds with concomitant peripheral disease	72	16 weeks	Twice/week	72.2% of patients had a rate of healing higher than 90%.
Anitua et al[26]	Randomised open-label controlled pilot trial	Chronic cutaneous ulcers	15 PRP: 8 patients Control : 7 patients	8 weeks	Once/week	Mean percentage of surface healed in the PRGF group was 72.94% +/- 22.25% compared to 21.48% +/- 33.56% in the control group [p < 0.05)
Sarvajnamurthy S et al[27]	Case series	Venous ulcers	12	6 weeks	Once/week	100% improvement in the volume of the ulcers was seen in 14 patients (82%). Mean percentage improvement in the area and volume of the ulcer was 94.7% and 95.6% respectively .No side effects were noted and there was a decrease in pain associated with the ulcers.
Suryanarayan et al[28]	Nonrandomized, uncontrolled study	Chronic non healing ulcers	24	6 weeks	Once/week	Mean percentage of improvement in area and volume of the ulcers was 91.7% and 95% respectively . Complete reduction in volume was seen in 73% of the ulcers by 6 weeks of treatment.
Saad setta et al[29]	comparative study	Chronic diabetic foot ulcers	24 Group A (n=12):PRP Group B (n=12):PPP	20 weeks	Twice/week	Mean healing time for PRP was 11·5 weeks and 17 weeks for PPP. Healing in PRP group was significantly faster (P < 0·005).

*ORC: oxidized regenerated cellulose; PPP: platelet-poor plasma

Other therapies

Platelet-rich fibrin (PRF) is a second-generation autologous leukocyte and platelet-rich concentrate incorporated within a fibrin matrix, prepared by simplified processing without the addition of anticoagulants. The fibrin matrix in PRF is the key element responsible for the real therapeutic potential of PRF.[30] The PRF membranes support the initiation of angiogenesis, accelerate healing, favour micro vascularization and guide epithelial cell migration.

Our experience

A 56-year-old diabetic male presented with a corn on the right little toe. The patient had underlying vitamin B12 and vitamin D deficiencies, and abnormal iron studies at the time of corn excision, which were simultaneously corrected. However, the patient developed a non-healing ulcer despite adequate treatment until two weeks post excision. Thereafter a single session of platelet-rich fibrin application was done, following which initiation of re-epithelization was noted within three days and complete re-epithelization was noted within two weeks of the procedures depicted in Figure 3.

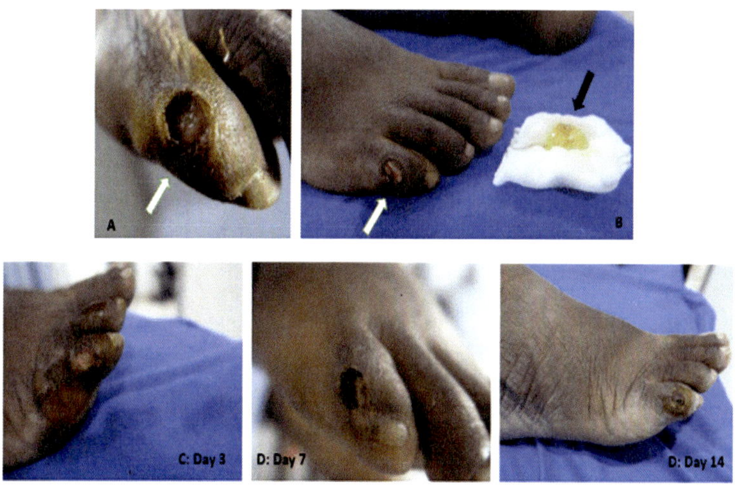

Figure 3: PRF membrane in non-healing ulcer post corn excision in a diabetic patient
*White arrow indicates non-healing ulcer; black arrow indicates platelet-rich fibrin
A: non-healing ulcer; B: PRF application; C: initiation of ulcer re-epithelization on day 3 post PRF; D: day 7 post PRF with crusted and epithelialized very shallow ulcer; E: ulcer re-epithelialized with superficial scab formation on day 14.

Combination or "cocktail" treatments

PRP and autologous fat graft

Adipose-derived stem cells are believed to facilitate healing through differentiation into cells that influence wound healing. Combinations with PRP increases survival of the fat graft due to early vascularization of the fat via the pro-angiogenic effects of PRP, therefore reversing the early ischaemic phase of the graft.[17] Cervelli et al. observed re-epithelization in 16 out of 20 patients with chronic lower-extremity ulcers who were treated with a combination of PRP and autologous fat graft, compared with 2 of 10 similar wounds treated with hyaluronic acid- and collagen-based medication.[31]

Platelet-rich plasma and mesenchymal stem cells

Stem cells play a significant role in the healing of chronic non-healing wounds by their properties of cellular differentiation, regeneration, immunomodulatory properties and the ability to release growth factors. Raposio et al. noted a higher rate of wound closure in the group treated with a single session of enriched PRP (PRP mixed with adipose tissue-derived stem cells) versus standard wound care therapy.[32]

Platelet-rich plasma (PRP) and hyaluronic acid (HA)

Hyaluronic acid aids in healing by regulating the tissue hydration and osmotic balance, and acts as a dermal substitute and a scaffold for the PRP. A combination of PRP and HA has been demonstrated to aid in epidermal proliferation and tissue regeneration.[33]

Cocktail of ablative Pixel erbium YAG laser, PRP therapy and autologous fat transplant

A twenty-eight-year-old male patient with a post-traumatic scar with recurrent trophic ulcers received a cocktail therapy of Pixel erbium YAG laser, PRP and autologous fat transplantation with which complete healing of the trophic ulcer and 40% improvement in touch and pain sensations over the heel was noted.[34]

Other combination therapies that have been tried are PRP with oxidized regenerated cellulose.[22]

Conclusion

Wound healing is a complex process and non-healing ulcers constitute significant morbidity among patients. Regenerative medicine is a new weapon in the armamentarium of wound healing treatment strategies wherein autologous growth factors are utilized. PRP, being an elixir of growth factors, is an innovative and a safe tool to accelerate the healing in chronic wounds.

References

1. Frykberg RG, Banks J. Challenges in the treatment of chronic wounds. *Adv Wound Care*. 2015 Sep 1;**4**:560-82.
2. Everts PAM, Knape JTA, Weibrich G, Schönberger JPAM, Hoffmann J, Overdevest EP, et al. Platelet-rich plasma and platelet gel: a review. *J Extra Corpor Technol*. 2006 Jun;**38**:174-87.
3. Schultz GS, Chin GA, Moldawer L, Diegelmann RF. Principles of wound healing. In: Fitridge R, Thompson M, editors. Mechanisms of vascular disease: a reference book for vascular specialists. Adelaide (AU): University of Adelaide Press; 2011 [no updated date; cited 25 February 2021] [Internet]. Available from: http://www.ncbi.nlm.nih.gov/books/ NBK534261/
4. Suthar M, Gupta S, Bukhari S, Ponemone V. Treatment of chronic non-healing ulcers using autologous platelet rich plasma: a case series. *J Biomed Sci*. 2017 Dec 1;**24**:16.
5. American College of Surgeons Division of Education: Blended surgical education and training for life®. Nonhealing_wounds. [Internet]. [no updated date; cited 23 February 2021]. Available from: https://www.facs.org/-/media/files/education/core-curriculum/ nonhealing_ wounds.ashx
6. Broughton G, Janis JE, Attinger CE. Wound healing: an overview. *Plast Reconstr Surg*. 2006 Jun;**117**(supplement):1e-S-32e-S.
7. Edwards R, Harding KG. Bacteria and wound healing. *Curr Opin Infect Dis*. 2004 Apr;**17**:91-6.
8. Wolcott RD, Rhoads DD, Dowd SE. Biofilms and chronic wound inflammation. *J Wound Care*. 2008 Aug;**17**:333-41.
9. Demidova-Rice TN, Hamblin MR, Herman IM. Acute and impaired wound healing: pathophysiology and current methods for drug delivery, part 1: normal and chronic wounds: biology, causes, and approaches to care. *Adv Skin Wound Care*. 2012 Jul;**25**:304-14.

10. Caley MP, Martins VLC, O'Toole EA. Metalloproteinases and wound healing. *Adv Wound Care*. 2015 Apr 1;**4**:225-34.
11. Nguyen TT, Mobashery S, Chang M. Roles of matrix metalloproteinases in cutaneous wound healing. In: Alexandrescu V, editor. Wound Healing – new insights into ancient challenges. London: IntechOpen 12 Oct 2016 [no updated date; cited 25 Feb 2021] [Internet]. Available from: https://www.intechopen.com/books/wound-healing-new-insights-into-ancient-challenges/roles-of-matrix-metalloproteinases-in-cutaneous-wound-healing
12. Dohan Ehrenfest DM, Andia I, Zumstein MA, Zhang C-Q, Pinto NR, Bielecki T. Classification of platelet concentrates (platelet-rich plasma – PRP, platelet-rich fibrin – PRF) for topical and infiltrative use in orthopaedic and sports medicine: current consensus, clinical implications and perspectives. *Muscles Ligaments Tendons J*. 2014 May 8;**4**:3-9.
13. Akingboye AA, Giddins S, Gamston P, Tucker A, Navsaria H, Kyriakides C. Application of autologous derived-platelet rich plasma gel in the treatment of chronic wound ulcer: diabetic foot ulcer. *J Extra Corpor Technol*. 2010 Mar;**42**:20-29.
14. Alves R, Grimalt R. A review of platelet-rich plasma: history, biology, mechanism of action, and classification *Skin Appendage Disord*. 2018 Jan;4:18-24. [no updated date; cited 25 Feb 2021] [Internet]. Available from: https://www.ncbi.nlm.nih.gov/pmc/articles/PMC5806188/
15. Knighton DR, Ciresi KF, Fiegel VD, Austin LL, Butler EL. Classification and treatment of chronic nonhealing wounds. Successful treatment with autologous platelet-derived wound healing factors (PDWHF). *Ann Surg*. 1986 Sep;**204**:322–30.
16. Martinez-Zapata MJ, Martí-Carvajal AJ, Solà I, Expósito JA, Bolíbar I, Rodríguez L, et al. Autologous platelet-rich plasma for treating chronic wounds. *Cochrane Database Syst Rev*. 2016 May 25;**2016**:CD006899.
17. Blanton MW, Hadad I, Johnstone BH, Mund JA, Rogers PI, Eppley BL, et al. Adipose stromal cells and platelet-rich plasma therapies synergistically increase revascularization during wound healing. *Plast Reconstr Surg*. 2009 Feb;**123**(2 Suppl.):56S-64S.
18. Anandan V, Jameela WA, Saraswathy P, Sarankumar S. Platelet rich plasma: efficacy in treating trophic ulcers in leprosy. *J Clin Diagn Res JCDR*. 2016 Oct;**10**:WC06–9.
19. Hu Z, Qu S, Zhang J, Cao X, Wang P, Huang S, et al. Efficacy and safety of platelet-rich plasma for patients with diabetic ulcers: a systematic review and meta-analysis. *Adv Wound Care*. 2019 Jul 1;8:298-308.

20. Ahmed M, Reffat SA, Hassan A, Eskander F. Platelet-rich plasma for the treatment of clean diabetic foot ulcers. *Ann Vasc Surg.* 2017 Jan;38:206-11.
21. Mohammadi MH, Molavi B, Mohammadi S, Nikbakht M, Mohammadi AM, Mostafaei S, et al. Evaluation of wound healing in diabetic foot ulcer using platelet-rich plasma gel: a single-arm clinical trial. *Transfus Apher Sci.* 2017 Apr;**56**:160-164.
22. Kakagia DD, Kazakos KJ, Xarchas KC, Karanikas M, Georgiadis GS, Tripsiannis G, et al. Synergistic action of protease-modulating matrix and autologous growth factors in healing of diabetic foot ulcers. A prospective randomized trial. *J Diabetes Complications.* 2007 Nov;**21**: 387-91.
23. Qu DS, Hu DZ, Zhang PY, Wang DP, Li DS, Huang DS, et al. Clinical studies on platelet-rich plasma (PRP) therapy for chronic cutaneous ulcers: a systematic review and meta-analysis of randomized controlled trials. 2021 [no updated date; cited 25 February 2021] [Internet]. Available from: https://www.liebertpub.com/doi/abs/10.1089/ wound.2020.1186
24. Jeong S-H, Han S-K, Kim W-K. Treatment of diabetic foot ulcers using a blood bank platelet concentrate. *Plast Reconstr Surg.* 2010 Mar;**125**:944-52.
25. Kontopodis N, Tavlas E, Papadopoulos G, Pantidis D, Kafetzakis A, healing of diabetic foot ulcers in patients with concomitant peripheral arterial disease and critical limb ischemia. *Int J Low Extrem Wounds.* 2016 Mar;**15**:45-51.
26. Anitua E, Aguirre JJ, Algorta J, Ayerdi E, Cabezas AI, Orive G, et al. Effectiveness of autologous preparation rich in growth factors for the treatment of chronic cutaneous ulcers. *J Biomed Mater Res B Appl Biomater.* 2008 Feb;**84B**:415-21.
27. Sarvajnamurthy S, Suryanarayan S, Budamakuntala L, Suresh DH. Autologous platelet rich plasma in chronic venous ulcers: study of 17 cases. *J Cutan Aesthetic Surg.* 2013;**6**:97-9.
28. Suryanarayan S, Budamakuntla L, Khadri SIS, Sarvajnamurthy S. Efficacy of autologous platelet-rich plasma in the treatment of chronic nonhealing leg ulcers. *Plast Aesthetic Res.* 2014 Aug 28;**1**:65-9.
29. Saad Setta H, Elshahat A, Elsherbiny K, Massoud K, Safe I. Platelet-rich plasma versus platelet-poor plasma in the management of chronic diabetic foot ulcers: a comparative study. *Int Wound J.* 2011 Jun;**8**:307-12.
30. Choukroun J, Diss A, Simonpieri A, Girard M-O, Schoeffler C, Dohan SL, et al. Platelet-rich fibrin (PRF): a second-generation platelet

concentrate. Part IV: clinical effects on tissue healing. *Oral Surg Oral Med Oral Pathol Oral Radiol Endod*. 2006 Mar;**101**:e56-60.
31. Cervelli V, Gentile P, Grimaldi M. Regenerative surgery: use of fat grafting combined with platelet-rich plasma for chronic lower-extremity ulcers. *Aesthetic Plast Surg*. 2009 May;**33**:340-5.
32. Raposio E, Bertozzi N, Bonomini S, Bernuzzi G, Formentini A, Grignaffini E, et al. Adipose-derived stem cells added to platelet-rich plasma for chronic skin ulcer therapy. *Wounds Compend Clin Res Pract*. 2016 Apr;**28**:126-31.
33. De Angelis B, D'Autilio MFLM, Orlandi F, Pepe G, Garcovich S, Scioli MG, et al. Wound healing: in vitro and in vivo evaluation of a bio-functionalized scaffold based on hyaluronic acid and platelet-rich plasma in chronic ulcers. *J Clin Med*. 2019 Sep 18;**8**:1486. doi: 10.3390/jcm8091486. PMID: 31540446; PMCID: PMC6780765.
34. Garg S. Post-traumatic scar with repeated trophic ulcers treated with a cocktail of ablative Pixel erbium YAG laser, PRP therapy and autologous fat transplant – a novel case report of terminal nerve ending regeneration through regenerative surgery. *J Mol Genet Med* 2017; **11** [no updated date; cited 26 March 2021] [Internet]. Available from: https://www.omicsonline.org/open-access/post-traumatic-scar-with-repeated-trophic-ulcers-treated-with-a-cocktail-of-ablative-pixel-erbium-yag-laser-prp-therapy-and-autolo-1747-0862-1000303-96128.html

CHAPTER 13

SIDE EFFECTS AND COMPLICATIONS OF PRP THERAPY

AAYUSHI SHAH, SHEFALI PORWAL, ANUVA BANSAL, SURUCHI GARG

Platelet-rich plasma (PRP) is an autologous preparation of plasma which has a platelet concentration about 3 to 5 times the baseline values. Plasma with a platelet concentration greater than 1,000,000 platelets/µl and at least 5 ml would qualify as PRP. This is the widely accepted working definition of PRP.[1]

Platelets contain over 800 proteins, including about 1,500 protein-based bioactive factors.[2] These consist of growth factors, peptides, chemo-attractants and bioactive molecules. Circulating platelets are usually in an inactive state; contact with both native and exogenous molecules activates them. Activators include collagen, platelet-activating factor, calcium, magnesium, adenosine diphosphate (ADP) and thrombin. Activation precipitates degranulation and bioactive molecules are released, which promote growth and healing in the surrounding tissue.[3]

Some of the common growth factors identified in PRP include epidermal growth factors (EGF), platelet-derived growth factors (PDGF), transforming growth factor – beta 1 (TGF-beta1), endothelial cell growth factor and basic fibroblast growth factor. These have been shown to promote epidermal cell growth and differentiation, angiogenesis, etc. Thus, the effects of PRP, which promote healing, are also mitogenic. This leads to the question – "Could PRP promote atypia and tumorigenesis?" Notably, however, the growth factors in PRP do not enter the cell or its nucleus; they only bind to the membrane receptors. From there, they transduce signals promoting repair and healing. Thus, PRP is *not* mutagenic and has an excellent safety profile.[4]

Concerns over transmission and promotion of infections with PRP

Being an autologous preparation, PRP is inherently safe. There is no risk of transmission of infections such as HIV or hepatitis B[5]. PRP also has a pH of 6.5 to 6.7, which has been found to inhibit microbial growth, thus reducing risk of secondary bacterial infections.[5]

Overall, there is a paucity of data regarding the occurrence of adverse effects with use of PRP in dermatology. However, most studies on PRP report minimal to nil long-term and serious adverse effects. The commonly reported side effects after a PRP treatment are summarized in Table 1.

Table 1: Types of complications seen after PRP treatment	
I	Complications during preparation • bruising at phlebotomy site • clotting of collected blood sample (improper usage of anticoagulant) • complications due to use of activator (burning)
II	Immediate side effects (during injection of PRP) • pain • burning sensation • pinpoint bleeding • erythema • hypersensitivity reactions/allergic reactions • vasovagal attacks
III	Short-term side effects (after injection of PRP) • bruising/ecchymosis • headache • protracted tenderness • swelling of injected area • skin sensitivity • bacterial infections • folliculitis • itching, dryness, desquamation • pyogenic granuloma
IV	Long-term side effects • scarring • discoloration of skin • blindness
V	Systemic side effects • hypersensitivity reactions
VI	Others • cross-labelling/mixing of samples • procedural delays • inability to achieve adequate concentration of platelets (failure of procedure)

Details of commonly encountered side effects, and how to manage them

Immediate side effects

Mild pain during administration: A majority of patients receiving PRP treatment will experience pain and discomfort during the procedure, in spite of a local anaesthetic application. Use of vibratory anaesthesia, local tapping and nerve blocks have all been advocated to improve patient comfort. In a study of PRP for androgenetic alopecia, 100% patients reported pain during the procedure, despite local anaesthesia.[6] Around 25% of the patients reported persistent pain after the procedure, which lasted up to four hours.[6] If topical anaesthesia is being used (generally preferred for PRP on the face), we recommend using a thick layer for more than one hour, under occlusion, to achieve adequate numbing of the skin. Injectable anaesthesia is recommended for PRP on the scalp, and use of a ring block or regional nerve blocks is recommended.

Burning sensation: In a study on the face and neck revitalization with PRP, burning was reported in 70% of patients for about three minutes after the procedure.[7] In another study for PRP given in the periorbital region, mild burning was reported by all the patients during the procedure.[8] The addition of calcium chloride as an activator may contribute to the burning. The authors do not recommend using an activator when PRP is being injected into the skin or scalp, as collagen acts as a natural activator.

Bleeding: Short-lasting pinpoint bleeding is seen in all patients while administering PRP. However, patients with bleeding diathesis, patients on blood thinners or anticoagulants for example are at risk for protracted bleeding, and these factors should be ruled out before planning the procedure.

Hypersensitivity reactions: These may occur due to human error such as cross-labelling of samples, or due to any of the additives or activators of PRP.

Mild erythema: Mild erythema will occur in all patients due to the injections, which resolves within 24 hours. Erythema was noted in 80% of patients when PRP was administered to the face by Redaelli et al.[7], which resolved without any further treatment.

Allergic reactions (such as an urticarial rash): There exists a single case report of an allergic rash occurring within two hours of administration of PRP for an orthopaedic indication.[9] The rash resolved within four days without further complications.

Fullness or tight feeling in the scalp: This may last up to one day.

Scalp sensitivity: This is reported by many patients during the first hair wash after taking scalp PRP. Increased hair fall lasting for one week is reported by many patients.

Transient oedema: This was reported by some subjects after PRP treatment.[10]

Short-term side effects

Bruising/ecchymosis: Bruising may occur, especially when PRP is administered to the face. Patients should be informed about this during the pre-procedure counselling. In the study by Redaelli et al. consisting of 23 patients, bruising was reported in 3% of patients.[7]

Headache: Some patients report a headache after PRP injections on the scalp, along with a feeling of tightening of the scalp. This usually lasts for 24 to 48 hours. Patients may be prescribed over-the-counter painkillers such as paracetamol to manage such pain but NSAIDs should be strictly avoided in case they knock off the growth factors.

Protracted tenderness and skin sensitivity: Patients should be warned about the possibility of such effects. It may be advisable to avoid a hair wash for the first 12–24 hours after a procedure. Application of facial creams and massages after face PRP should be avoided for 48 hours. This will help to reduce the discomfort.

Swelling of injected area: Swelling of the areas where PRP is injected, or the area where nerve block is administered prior to PRP, may last for 24–48 hours. Figure 1 depicts such an image of a swelling on the forehead seen after injection of local anaesthetic.

Bacterial infections: Folliculitis, furunculosis and similar may occur at injection sites if proper asepsis is not followed, or in patients predisposed to infections (diabetics, immunosuppression, etc.) or with pre-existing infections elsewhere in the body. Antibiotic prophylaxis should be considered on a case-by-case basis.

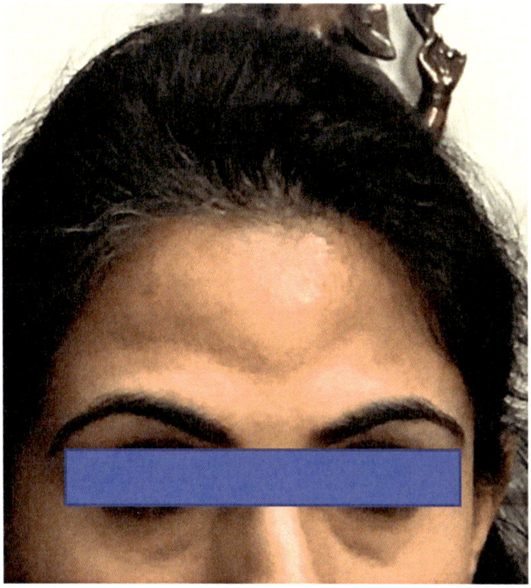

Figure 1: Self-limiting post-procedure swelling over forehead due to ring block (PRP therapy for female pattern hair loss).

Itching, dryness and desquamation of injected skin: These are common side effects occurring for a few days after PRP, on the face as well as the scalp. Adequate hydration before and after the procedure may be preventive.

Pyogenic granuloma: This has been reported as a side effect in a case after LA-PEEST (laser ablation of the recipient area with PRP-enriched epidermal suspension transplant) therapy for a vitiligo patch.[11] This could be explained by the increased vascularity seen after PRP injections due to the presence of VEGF in the PRP concentrate. Cases have also been seen after using PRP for other indications, such as in combination with hair transplant.

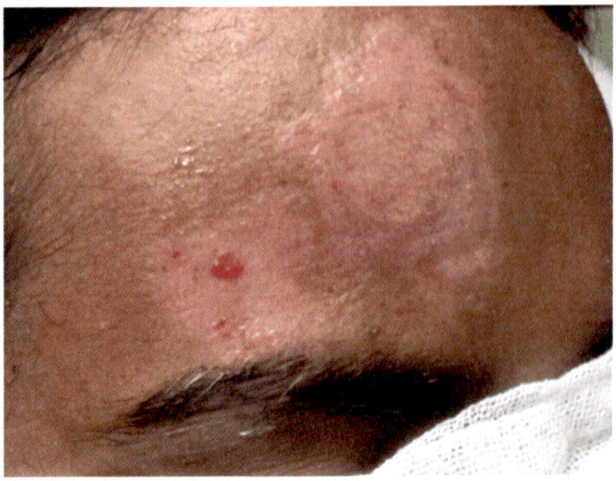

Figure 2: Pyogenic granuloma-like lesion seen two weeks after laser ablation over recipient area with PRP-enriched epidermal suspension transplant (LA-PEEST) for segmental vitiligo over forehead. Photo: Dr Suruchi Garg, Aura Skin Institute, Chandigarh.

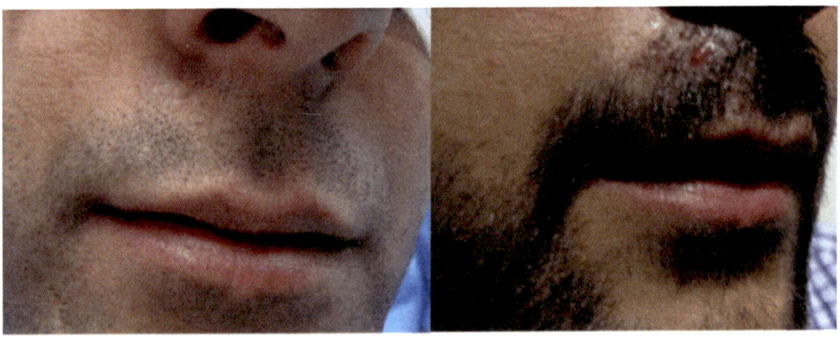

Figure 3: Pyogenic granuloma-like lesion two weeks after follicular unit extraction (FUE) hair transplant and PRP therapy for treatment of scarring alopecia. Photo: Dr Suruchi Garg, Aura Skin Institute, Chandigarh.

Long-term side effects

Scarring: This is secondary to deeper bacterial infections.

Discoloration of skin: Blood mixed with PRP due to faulty techniques of preparation, when administered, may give rise to pigmentation due to haemosiderin deposition at the sites of injection.

Blindness: There has been one case report of irreversible long-term blindness occurring in a 49-year-old woman, immediately following injection of autologous PRP in the glabellar region for rhytides[12]. This was accompanied by an area of ecchymosis and induration above the right medial eyebrow. Visual loss occurred due to acute right ophthalmic artery occlusion and brain infarction following autologous PRP injection. Histopathology from the site showed giant cell reactions for lipid-based foreign bodies. This was hypothesized to be due to inappropriate pre-mixing of fillers or fat with PRP along with an inadvertent intra-arterial injection by an unqualified practitioner[12]. The authors strongly advise against the pre-mixing of PRP with any other products, to maintain the inherent safety of the procedure.

A recent case series has evaluated four patients treated by cosmetologists with PRP injections who developed irreversible blindness due to iatrogenic occlusion of the ophthalmic artery. This happened immediately after the injection in the glabellar area in three cases and in the nasolabial fold in one case. The glabella is one of the most susceptible areas to tissue necrosis due its vascular anatomy (small vessels branching from supratrochlear and supraorbital arteries with limited collateral circulation).[13]

Systemic side effects

Risk of transmission of infections: This does not exist with PRP as PRP is an autologous preparation.

Hypersensitivity reactions: These are rarely known to occur. There is one report of an urticarial reaction occurring after PRP administration, which resolved within 4 days.[9]

Others

Methodical errors: Errors typically include the following:

- *Cross-labelling/mixing of samples* – these may lead to fatal hypersensitivity reactions, as well as a serious risk of transmission of blood-borne infections. Meticulous labelling is essential during every procedure. It is also advisable to avoid performing multiple procedures at the same time.

- *Procedural delays* – activation of platelets occurs mainly before injection; if there is a delay in using the PRP after its preparation, this could lead to a loss in the efficacy of the procedure. The PRP must always be injected immediately upon preparation.

- *Inability to achieve adequate platelet concentration* – this is usually due to incorrect technique employed during PRP preparation and centrifugation, and leads to a poor outcome of procedure.

Needle prick injuries to health practitioners: The risks involved with PRP are the same as with any invasive procedure. Hence, the procedure and handling of blood products should only be performed by trained and qualified medical professionals, and universal precautions must be followed at every step. Use of gloves, mask and eye protection is a must when performing the procedure.

Complications related to exogenous additives to PRP/ platelet activators

PRP by itself is immunologically neutral and poses no danger of allergy, hypersensitivity or reactions to foreign bodies when administered as an autologous preparation. However, any modifications done to the PRP increase the risk for allergic and hypersensitivity reactions, and such practices should be avoided. Collagen in skin and soft tissue is a natural activator of PRP, so when PRP is used in soft tissue, it does not need to be exogenously activated[14]. The following are the existing reports of adverse effects with some of the commonly used PRP activators.

Calcium chloride

Calcium chloride is commonly added before injection of PRP to promote activation of platelets and the release of growth factors. There has been a single case report of an allergic rash upon intralesional PRP administration for a tibial bone cyst, in which calcium chloride used for activation was the cause of a type 1 hypersensitivity reaction[9]. The skin rash appeared within the first 24 hours of receiving the PRP injection. The clinicians reported small red papular, purpuric eruptions predominantly on the extremities. Testing with intradermal calcium citrate was positive. Patient was treated with antihistamines and symptoms were alleviated in four days.

Use of xenogeneic thrombin (bovine thrombin) as an activator

Exogenous bovine thrombin is used in certain methods of preparation of PRP for orthopaedic indications. However, thrombin is not routinely used for activation of PRP in dermatological indications. The use of bovine thrombin has reportedly been associated with the development of antibodies to human clotting factors V, XI and thrombin, resulting in a risk of potentially life-threatening coagulopathies in a few case reports. Also, bovine thrombin has a completely negative history for transmission of Creutzfeldt-Jakob disease (mad cow disease) as was earlier thought; however, that risk has now completely been refuted.[5]

Basal cell carcinoma

There is a single case reported from France of two basal cell carcinomas occurring in a 79-year-old woman, eight months after having received a PRP injection procedure for facial rejuvenation[15]. However, considering the age of the patient and history of significant sun exposure, a direct causative relationship to the PRP injections could not be established. The patient claimed not to have the cutaneous lesions prior to having received the PRP treatment. The authors of this case report have called for further studies on the safety of PRP and vigilance by all practitioners.

Contraindications to PRP treatment

Absolute contraindications

- haemodynamic instability
- platelet defects
- septicaemia
- anticoagulant therapy
- hypofibrinogenemia
- local infections

Relative contraindications

- chronic liver and kidney disease
- recent use of NSAIDs (in the past 72 hours)
- recent use of systemic steroids (in the past 15 days)
- severe anaemia
- unstable angina

Suggested measures to avoid side effects during PRP therapy

- Maintain sterility of all equipment.
- Use a dedicated centrifuge at point-of-care to avoid mixing of samples and delays in administration.
- Labelling of samples is of utmost importance to avoid sampling errors. All staff should be well trained in this.
- Use only freshly prepared autologous PRP for optimal efficacy.
- Avoid the use of external additives and activators as much as possible. This automatically eliminates the risk of many adverse effects (in dermatological indications no activators are required, as PRP is injected in soft tissue, with collagen being a natural activator).
- Universal precautions should be used for all injectors and handlers throughout the procedure.
- Rule out thrombocytopenia, platelet defects and systemic illnesses before considering the procedure.
- Intradermal sensitivity testing may be performed prior to the procedure in cases with a history of urticaria or past episodes of hypersensitivity.
- Preparation and administration of PRP should be done only by doctors or registered medical practitioners.
- Use appropriate anaesthesia to reduce procedural pain.
- Keep an emergency kit available at all times in the procedure room.
- Provide adequate patient counselling regarding short-term transient side effects such as headache, pain, sensitivity and management of the same.

There are many studies elaborating the positive outcome of PRP; however, negative aspects are yet to be explored further. According to one proposition, the response of cells to an external environment, such as being subjected to high-speed centrifugation, cannot be predicted. The cells may behave differently, compared to when they are in their "natural environment". The platelets, when injected, can also disseminate instead of being localized at the injection site, resulting in untoward side effects.[16]

The effect on the body of anticoagulants and activators used in the preparation of PRP remains to be studied in scientific trials, especially after the COVID-19 times. Although decades of clinical experience have demonstrated it to be a safe therapy, scientific data is still lacking. Therefore, an appropriate selection of patients before considering the procedure and detailed pre-procedure counselling is of utmost importance.

There should be a pre-treatment haematologic evaluation, and unsuitable candidates should be eliminated from treatments.

Long-term randomized clinical trials are much needed to establish the downstream effects of this therapy.

PRP in the COVID scenario

The COVID-19 related hypercoagulable state may theoretically increase the risk of inadvertent arterial occlusion and subsequent complications resulting from the accidental intra-arterial injection of PRP.

Although PRP is an autologous cell therapy, it contains a high concentration of live platelets, growth factors, cytokines, chemokines and proteins, which exert a plethora of paracrine, autocrine and enzymatic effects, the complete influence of which remains a mystery.

Hence, it may be deemed as "a mighty dragon warrior" to be used with the utmost caution, especially around periorbital, glabellar and mid-face areas.[17,18]

References

1. Marx RE. Platelet-rich plasma (PRP): What is PRP and what is not PRP? *Implant Dent.* 2001;**10**:225-8.
2. Boswell SG, Cole BJ, Sundman EA, Karas V, Fortier LA. Platelet-rich plasma: a milieu of bioactive factors. *Arthroscopy.* 2012 Mar;**28**:429-39.
3. Foster TE, Puskas BL, Mandelbaum BR, Gerhardt MB, Rodeo SA. Platelet-rich plasma: from basic science to clinical applications. *Am J Sports Med.* 2009;**37**:2259-2272.
4. Schmitz JP, Hollinger JO. The biology of platelet-rich plasma. *J Oral Maxillofac Surg.* 2001;**59**:1119-21.
5. Choi J, Minn KW, Chang H. The efficacy and safety of platelet-rich plasma and adipose-derived stem cells: an update. *Arch Plast Surg.* 2012 Nov;**39**:585-92.
6. Gkini MA, Kouskoukis AE, Tripsianis G, Rigopoulos D, Kouskoukis K. Study of platelet-rich plasma injections in the treatment of androgenetic alopecia through a one-year period. *J Cutan Aesthet Surg* 2014;**7**:213-9.
7. Redaelli A, Romano D, Marcianó A. Face and neck revitalization with platelet-rich plasma (PRP): clinical outcome in a series of 23 consecutively treated patients. *J Drugs Dermatol.* 2010 May;**9**:466-72.

8. Mehryan P, Zartab H, Rajabi A, Pazhoohi N, Firooz A. Assessment of efficacy of platelet-rich plasma (PRP) on infraorbital dark circles and crow's feet wrinkles. *J Cosmet Dermatol*. 2014 Mar;**13**:72-8.
9. Latalski M, Walczyk A, Fatyga M, Rutz E, Szponder T, Bielecki, T. et al. Allergic reaction to platelet-rich plasma (PRP): Case report. *Medicine (Baltimore)*. 2019 Mar;**98**:e14702.
10. Cervantes J, Perper M, Wong LL, Eber AE, Villasante Fricke AC, Wikramanayake TC, et al. Effectiveness of platelet-rich plasma for androgenetic alopecia: a review of the literature. *Skin Appendage Disord*. 2018 Jan;**4**:1-11.
11. Garg S, Dosapaty N, Arora AK. Laser ablation of the recipient area with platelet-rich plasma–enriched epidermal suspension transplant in vitiligo surgery: a pilot study. *Dermatol Surg* 2019 Jan;**45**:83-89. doi: 10.1097/DSS.0000000000001641.
12. Kalyam K, Kavoussi SC, Ehrlich M, Teng CC, Chadha N, Khodadadeh S, et al. Irreversible blindness following periocular autologous platelet-rich plasma skin rejuvenation treatment. *Ophthalmic Plast Reconstr Surg*. 2017 May/Jun;**33**(3S Suppl. 1):S12-S16.
13. Karam EZ, Gan A, Muci Mendoza R, Martinez E, Perez E. Visual loss after platelet-rich plasma injection into the face. *Neuroophthalmology*. 2020;**44**:371-378.
14. Dhurat R, MS Sukesh. Principles and methods of preparation of platelet-rich plasma: a review and author's perspective. *J Cutan Aesthet Surg*. 2014 Oct-Dec;**7**:189-197.
15. Dauendorffer JN, Fraitag S, Dupuy A. Basal cell carcinoma following platelet-rich plasma injection for skin rejuvenation. *Ann Dermatol Venereol*. 2013 Nov;**140**:723-4. doi: 10.1016/j.annder.2013.07.010.
16. Middleton KK, Barro V, Muller B, Terada S, Fu FH. Evaluation of the effects of platelet-rich plasma (PRP) therapy involved in the healing of sports-related soft tissue injuries. *Iowa Orthop J*. 2012;**32**:150.
17. Garg S. Regeneration through platelet rich plasma – a cell therapy with a path full of milestones, controversies and cautions! *Indian Dermatol Online J*. 2021 Nov 25;**12**(Suppl. 1):S1–3.
18. Garg S, Bansal A. Platelet-rich plasma in interventional dermatology and trichology: how far have we come? CSDM. 2021 Jun 10; [no updated date; cited 19 Apr 2022 19] [Internet]. Available from: https://cosmoderma.org/platelet-rich-plasma-in-interventional-dermatology-and-trichology-how-far-have-we-come/

CHAPTER 14

THE FUTURE OF REGENERATIVE MEDICINE AWAITS THE COCKTAIL OF VARIOUS LIVE CELLS

ANUVA BANSAL, SURUCHI GARG

Introduction

Stem cell therapies hold a promising place in the future of regenerative medicine with widespread therapeutic implications. Stem cells are undifferentiated cells present in different organ systems with the three hallmark characteristics of self-renewal, differentiation and plasticity. Stem cells are present in a specialized micro-environment called stem cell niche, which functions as a unit to maintain homeostasis and repair tissues at the time of injury.[1-3]

Stem cells can be classified on the basis of their source and differentiating capacity. In skin, they are present in the interfollicular epidermis, hair follicle, dermis and adipose tissue, which help in maintaining normal skin homeostasis, and repair and regeneration during injury.[4-7]

Although several clinical trials are investigating the safety and efficacy of stem cell therapies for the treatment of several dermatological conditions, additional basic and clinical research will need to be performed before stem cell therapy can become a mainstream treatment option and until then, platelet-rich plasma (PRP) therapy with its regenerative and regrowth potential in a plethora of conditions can be utilized along with stem cell suspension as a cocktail of live cells, for longer-lasting results with more sustainable effects.

Properties of stem cells

Stem cells have a number of properties such as self-renewal, differentiation and plasticiy,[2,8] the main ones being as follows:

1. Self-renewal: the ability to undergo numerous cycles of asymmetrical cell division to produce differentiated cells as well as cells that are similar to the parent cell, thereby maintaining the pool of undifferentiated cells.
2. Differentiation: the ability to differentiate into cells of the tissue in which the stem cell is located.
3. Plasticity/trans-differentiation: the ability of adult stem cells to cross lineage barriers and differentiate into cells of tissue different from the original tissue.

Based on their regeneration ability, stem cells can be classified into:

- totipotent cells, which can differentiate into all cell lineages and embryonic tissue;
- pluripotent cells, which can differentiate into all the three germ cell lineages, but not into extra-embryonic tissue;
- multipotent stem cells, which can differentiate into different cells of the same lineage;
- monopotent cells – as the name indicates – can regenerate only one cell type.

Classification of stem cells

Stem cells can be classified on the basis of their source and differentiating capacity. In skin, they are present in the interfollicular epidermis, hair follicle, dermis and adipose tissue. [1,4-7,9]

Cutaneous stem cells			
Type	Location	Marker	Properties
Hair follicle stem cells	The bulge region of the hair follicle, defined as the portion of the outer root sheath of the hair follicle at the insertion site of the arrector pili muscle	Cytokeratin 15	Injury to the epidermis results in migration of the bulge cells to the epidermis where they then contribute to wound repair. Golden anchorage aids in • hair follicle formation in the anagen phase • follicular integrity and survival
Melanocyte stem cells	Population of follicular bulge stem cells committed to melanocyte differentiation	Pax3, MITF	Melanocyte stem cells are usually quiescent but become activated and proliferate at the onset of the anagen phase. This leads to the repopulation of the hair follicle matrix with melanocytes that generate melanin leading to pigmentation of the hair shaft.
Sebaceous gland progenitor cells	Sebaceous glands	Blimp-1 (B lymphocyte-induced maturation protein-1)	Sebaceous gland homeostasis necessitates the presence of a progenitor population of cells that gives rise to a continual flux of proliferating, differentiating and disintegrating sebocytes.

Stem cells in the interfollicular epidermis	Basal layer, basement membrane, rete ridges, tip of dermal papillae. Each epidermal proliferative unit consists of a single centrally located stem cell, its immediate transient amplifying cell progeny adjacent, with more differentiated keratinocytes lying directly above and mature, enucleated, squamous cells at the surface.	Alpha 8-integrin, beta 1-integrin and CK15, CK10, CD71 desmosomal proteins	The interfollicular epidermis is dependent on multiple, functionally independent, hexagonal units called the epidermal proliferative units (EPU). These EPU ensure lifelong cell production to compensate for the continual loss of cells from the surface of the skin.
Sweat gland stem cells	Sweat glands	Nestin	Sweat gland renewal, homeostasis
Skin mesenchymal stem cells (MSCs)	Dermis and its components, adipose tissue in subcutis	CD44, CD73, CD90, CD105, CD166, Vimentin	MSCs are able to differentiate into adipocytes, osteocytes, chondrocytes, smooth muscle cells and haematopoietic supportive stroma. In a steady state or in response to injury, turnover of stromal tissue occurs through the participation of a population of stem cells found in the stromal tissue.
Adipose tissue-derived stem cells (AdSCs)	Adipose tissue	CD13, CD29, CD44, CD71, CD90, CD166	Activates the epithelial stem cells by secreting various growth factors. Hair follicles are surrounded by subcutis and dermis. Interfollicular epidermis forms a macro environment and promotes signalling mechanisms, which help in the maintenance of follicular stem cell reserve in the bulge region.

Role in regenerative medicine

Androgenetic alopecia (AGA)

Androgenetic alopecia (AGA) is associated with progressive miniaturization of the hair follicles (HFs) and a continuous reduction in the duration of the anagen phase with each cycle, producing microscopic hairs.

Current data indicates that human HFs also contain multipotent stem cells located in the bulge area, which can help in reversing the pathological mechanisms contributing to hair loss and can cause the regeneration of hair follicles through a process known as neogenesis. This knowledge is being utilized in the management of AGA where follicular suspension, containing stem cells alone or in combination with platelet-rich plasma (PRP), has produced favourable results.[10-12] Occipital hair, which is resistant to hormonal influences in androgenetic alopecia, is considered the best source for extraction of stem cells.[13]

In addition to replacing damaged cells in affected tissues, stem cells have beneficial effects through a paracrine action via various cytokines and growth factors. Hair regrowth is regulated primarily by ERK activation and Wnt signalling. Secretory factors derived from ADSCs include PDGF, hepatocyte growth factor (HGF), VEGF and IGF binding protein precursors, and fibronectin. PDGF has been shown to induce and maintain the anagen phase in the hair cycle in a mouse model while HGF facilitates hair follicle elongation. VEGF increases hair growth and size by follicle vascularization, and IGF-1 improves the migration, survival and proliferation of hair follicle cells.[14,15]

Recent studies have evaluated the effect of autologous stem cell suspension in patients with AGA, and have observed significant improvement in hair density compared to placebo or PRP alone. (Table 2)

Table 2: Studies evaluating the effect of autologous stem cell suspension in patients with AGA

Study	Groups	Intervention	Results
Gentile et al.[12]	11 patients with AGA	Autologous hair follicle stem cell (AFSC) suspension V/S placebo	$29 \pm 5\%$ increase in the hair density in the treatment group compared to $< 1\%$ in the group treated with the placebo
Kadry et al.[16]	60 patients with AGA	Three monthly sessions of either autologous adipose tissue-derived stem cell (ADSC) or platelet-rich plasma (PRP) therapy	Mean increase in hair density as evaluated by an increase in the terminal and intermediate hair count was significantly higher compared to baseline in the group treated with adipose tissue-derived stem cells ($p<0.001$ and $p<0.001$ respectively).
Tak et al.[17]	38 patients with AGA	Twice daily self-application of the adipose-derived stem cell constituent extract (ADSC-CE) topical solution over the scalp with fingers in the intervention group (IG) or to a control group (CG).	Phototrichogram at week 8 showed more increase in hair count in the IG than in the CG, and intergroup differences in the change of hair count remained significant until week 16 with overall changes of 28.1% vs 7.1%, respectively. Significant improvement in hair diameter was observed in the IG (14.2%) after 16 weeks when compared with hair diameter in the CG (6.3%).

Elmaadawi et al.[18]	20 patients with AGA	Patients were divided into two groups: • 10 AGA patients received a single session of intradermal injections of autologous bone marrow-derived mononuclear cells (BMMCs). • 10 AGA patients received a single session of follicular stem cells (FSC).	The mean percentage of improvement was: • 2± 28 in subjects receiving autologous BMMC; • 2± 27 in AGA subjects receiving autologous FSC with non-statistically significant differences. Both groups showed significant improvement with digital dermoscopy examination: • here was an increase in hair width, as well as hair density after six months of single SC injection therapy in all groups of patients. • ncreased immunoreactivities with CK15, CD34 and CD200 in all treated groups, which suggests that the stem cells were able to progress to hair germs and subsequent hair follicle organogenesis.

PRP with stem cell suspension

In our experience, a patient with AGA who had received five sessions of platelet-rich plasma was administered a single session of autologous hair follicle suspension (AFSC) comprising stem cells along with extracellular matrix admixed with platelet-rich plasma at a gap of six months from the last PRP session.

Fifty follicular unit grafts are extracted from the occipital area of the scalp (known to be resistant in androgenetic alopecia, thus an ideal source) and mixed with 5 ml of 0.25% trypsin EDTA solution. The solution containing grafts is incubated at a temperature of 40°C for two hours with frequent shaking. Later, it is mechanically agitated, filtered and centrifuged at 3,200 rpm for 10 minutes. The supernatant is discarded, the pellet formed is mixed with 5 ml of platelet-poor plasma and subjected to a second centrifugation at 3,200 rpm for 10 minutes. After discarding the supernatant, the lower portion of the solution along with the pellet is mixed with platelet-rich plasma to produce a uniform suspension. It is then transferred into a 1 ml insulin syringe and 0.05 ml is injected at 1 cm intervals in the androgen-sensitive area.

A follicular stem cell suspension comprising stem cells along with extracellular matrix combined with PRP was compared to PRP alone. The following was noted on clinical evaluation:

- a noticeable improvement in the texture of hair;
- a filling effect in the frontotemporal angles;
- relative increases in the proportion of course, terminal hair;
- improvement in the hairline, better with autologous hair follicle suspension compared to PRP therapy.

Videomicroscopy revealed multiple coarse, terminal and secondary hair sprouting along with primary follicular units after autologous stem cell transplant.

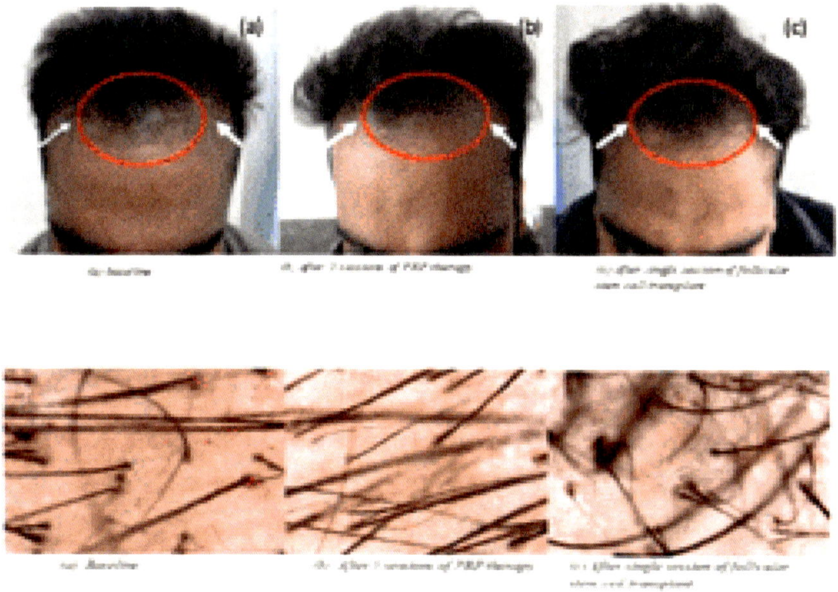

Figure 1: Use of follicular stem cells after five sessions of PRP therapy. Progressive change in the hairline is evident and video microscopy reveals increased and thicker hair follicles after PRP therapy, whereas sprouting of secondary and tertiary hair units after follicular suspension. Photo: S Garg[1]

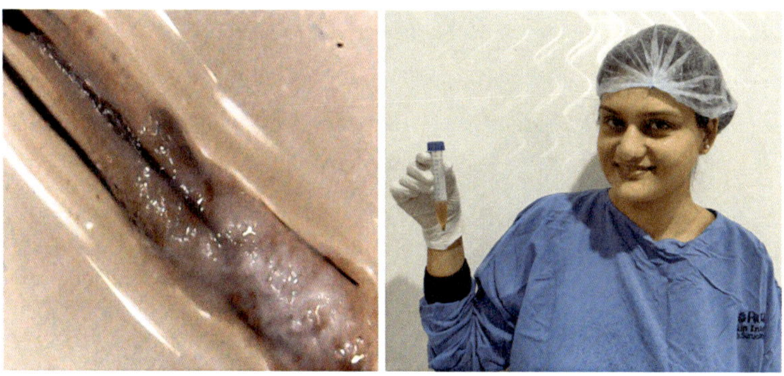

Figure 2: Trypsinized hair follicle graft after two hours of incubation showing bulge portion with secondary hair follicular unit under trichoscopy and first-time successful isolation of follicular stem cells admixed with PRP. Photo: Dr Suruchi Garg, Aura Skin Institute, Chandigarh, India.

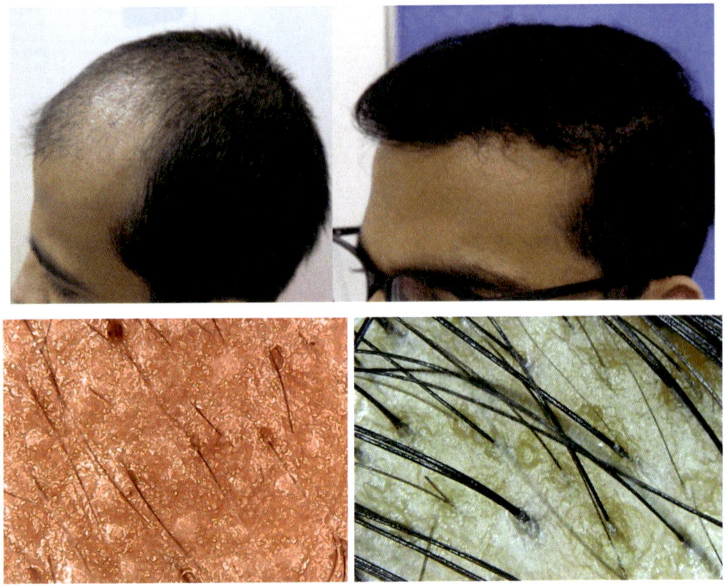

Figure 3: Clinical and trichoscopic images of a cocktail of FUE hair transplant with follicular suspension PRP therapy at baseline and four months later, managed with conventional multivitamin supplements, early morning plant-based protein, topical 5% minoxidil and peptide solution after the transplant. Trichoscopic images clearly show baseline vellus hair transforming into thicker intermediate hair along with sprouting of secondary units, alongside thick transplanted hair. Photo: Dr Suruchi Garg, Aura Skin Institute, Chandigarh, India.

The authors also compared the effect of PRP injections combined with follicular unit extraction (FUE) (Group 1) versus a combination of PRP, FUE, and follicular suspension (Group 2), among two groups of 40 men with AGA, in a comparative study (unpublished at the time of writing). Significantly more patients achieved greater than 75% hair density in Group 2 versus Group 1. Similarly, activity in dormant follicles as fine vellus hair later transforming into intermediate hair alongside the thick transplanted hair was seen starting as early as two months in the PRP plus FS group in all 20 patients compared to the non-FS group. In PRP group on the other hand, the start of this activity was seen in 14 patients three months onwards, not as perceivable at the end of one year. In the FS plus PRP-treated group, the number of patients having multiple grafts was significantly higher compared to the only PRP-treated group. Additionally, the length of hair shafts, texture and smoothness was superior compared to the other group.

Alopecia areata

Stem cells exhibit anti-inflammatory and immunomodulatory properties, in addition to stimulating hair growth. MSCs act by inhibiting the proliferation of T-cells and B-cells, and modify the function of other immune cells These cells have also been demonstrated to increase the secretion of immunosuppressive molecules such as IDO, PGE2 and TGF-β1, inhibit the maturation of dendritic cells (DCS), cause the upregulation of the JAK1/ STAT3 pathway and induce the differentiation of regulatory T-cells (Treg).[19-21]

Recent studies have evaluated the role of MSCs in the management of resistant and non-responsive cases of alopecia areata (AA).

In an open-labelled pilot study, the efficacy of follicular stem cell suspension was evaluated in eight patients with AA. Excellent (>50%) improvement was noted in 62.5% of patients, good (10–50%) improvement in 25% patients, and poor (<10%) improvement in one patient was observed at the end of six months of treatment.[19]

A retrospective study of 20 patients with AA used autologous stromal vascular fraction and demonstrated increased hair growth and decreased pull-test values three and six months after the therapy [hair density (85.1 ± 8.7 vs 121.1 ± 12.5 hair/cm^2, $P<0.0001$); hair diameter (60.5 ± 1.8 vs 80.8 ± 2.4μ, $P<0.0001$) and pull-test values (4.4 ± 0.3 vs 0.8 ± 0.2, $P<0.0001$), untreated versus six months post-operative)][20]

Another study compared the effect of intradermal injection of bone marrow-derived mononuclear cells (BMMCs) versus intradermal injections of autologous follicular stem cells (AFSC) in two groups of 10 patients with AA. Gradual improvement started by the end of the first month and reached its maximum improvement after six months, with no statistically significant difference between the methods. The patchy and the ophiasis types showed the highest response to SC therapy compared to alopecia totalis types. Increased immunoreactivities with CK 15, CD34 and CD200 suggested that the stem cells were able to progress to hair germs and subsequent hair follicle organogenesis, confirming the effectiveness of stem cell therapy in AA.[8]

Wound healing

Stem cell therapy has recently emerged as a promising treatment modality, with the potential to restore tissue to its pre-traumatic state and accelerate wound healing by modifying the immune response and promoting angiogenesis.[22]

Chronic wounds are defined as those that have failed to proceed through a systematic and timely reparative process and recent research has demonstrated that fibroblasts derived from chronic wounds resemble aged or senescent fibroblasts in vitro, and have reduced proliferation and impaired response to growth factors important for wound healing.[23]

Stem cells secrete cytokines and growth factors involved in immunomodulation and regeneration, making them a promising agent for correcting the underlying biological deficiencies observed in chronic wounds and have been explored for their ability to promote wound healing in several animal models and clinical trials. (Tables 3a and 3b)

Currently, the majority of stem cell-based trials for wound healing are utilizing mesenchymal stem cell-based interventions.

Table 3a: Types and sources of stem cells for wound healing

Type	Source	Advantages	Drawbacks
Embryonic stem cells (ESCs) [24,25]	ESCs are isolated from the inner cell mass of the blastocyst	Readily expandable in culture, and can be guided with growth factors in supplemented media to differentiate into mature cells involved in wound repair ESCs have been successfully differentiated into functional keratinocytes to form an epidermal sheet in vitro that could be used as a temporary skin substitute in patients awaiting autologous grafts	Ethical considerations and legal restrictions have limited the clinical use of ESCs.
Bone marrow-derived mesenchymal stem cells [26,27] (BM-MSCs)	Isolated from bone marrow	BM-MSCs have been shown to increase migration of fibroblasts and keratinocytes Enhances angiogenesis by increasing levels of vascular endothelial growth factor (VEGF) and hepatocyte growth factor (HGF) May initiate an inflammatory response in wounds that is favourable to healing outcomes	A significant barrier to clinical use of BM-MSC is their isolation, which requires obtaining bone marrow aspirates, a procedure that can cause significant patient morbidity and yield an insufficient number of cells required for treatment.

Adipose stem cells (ASCs) [28,29]	Isolated from lipoaspirates that are frequently disposed of as medical waste following procedures	ASC isolation from adipose tissue yields a high number of cells and allows clinical application without in vitro expansion. Resulting in accelerated healing and increased neovascularization of the wound	Collection of the tissue does not cause donor morbidity and is often discarded as medical waste.
Other MSC sources [30]	Human umbilical cord blood (UCB) and extra-foetal tissue, including amniotic fluid, Wharton's jelly, placental tissue and umbilical cord-lining tissue	Significant therapeutic potential Significant improvement in the rate and quality of wound healing	Collection of the tissue does not cause donor morbidity and is often discarded as medical waste.

Table 3b: Methods of stem cell application for wound healing

Method of stem cell application	Technique and advantages	Drawbacks
Local application		
Direct injection into or proximal to the wound [31]	A straightforward approach that has achieved significant improvement in wound healing	Cell survival, retention and engraftment are limited, likely due to mechanical disruption of the cell membrane as it passes through a syringe needle
Fibrin polymer spray system comprising MSC containing fibrinogen and thrombin[32]	Significantly decreased wound size and increased vascularity in diabetic mice	Not always possible due its invasiveness.
Microspheres and hydrophobic scaffolds [33,34]	Microsphere as a microcarrier for MSCs, achieving increased engraftment and retention and increased viability	No adverse effects
Hydrogels[35]	Can mimic a functional stem cell niche for the delivery of MSCs into wounds. MSCs within the hydrogels exhibited enhanced viability, engraftment and secretion of angiogenic cytokines, and expression of transcription factors.	-

Intravenous infusion[36]	An alternative method of stem cell delivery in instances where the site of injury is inaccessible, or a systemic therapeutic response is necessary. Immunomodulatory effects may be beneficial for wound healing.	The majority of infused cells are entrapped in pulmonary capillaries immediately after systemic infusion and exhibit limited migration beyond the lung, resulting in few cells reaching their target site.
Genetic engineering [37,38]	Retroviral/lentiviral and non-integrating viral vector, plasmid DNA, and mRNA transfection and nanoparticle delivery transduction.	Limited in their clinical application as viral delivery poses a high risk of oncogenic insertional mutagenesis and non-viral delivery of plasmids is not preserved as cells propagate

Post-traumatic and post-burn scars

Recent studies have demonstrated significant improvement in post-burn scars following both autologous lipografting and MSC application in terms of reduced Vancouver Scar Scale scores and clinical appearance.

Similar to growth factors released by PRP, MSCs are capable of promoting the renewal processes through augmenting angiogenesis as well as creating an anti-inflammatory and anti-fibrotic milieu. Lipofilling and adipose MSCs have been shown to lessen the risk of developing, as well as pre-existent fibrotic scarring.[39]

Forming new skin (enhancing healing by secondary intention): cocktail of live cells and PRP

Although several clinical trials are investigating the safety and efficacy of stem cell therapies for the treatment of burns and chronic wounds, additional basic and clinical research will need to be performed before stem cell therapy can become a mainstream treatment option.

Authors have innovated two procedures that utilize epidermal fragments, thus making use of epidermal stem cells enhanced with the presence of PRP growth factors to formulate new skin. This technique is called a PRP-enriched epidermal suspension transplant. When done in addition to ablative laser it is called LA-PEEST (laser ablation of recipient area with PRP-enriched epidermal suspension transplant) and when radiofrequency ablation of recipient area is done it is termed RA-PEEST (radiofrequency ablation on recipient area with PRP – enriched epidermal suspension transplant).

According to the author's experience, a cocktail of radiofrequency ablation, PRP-enriched trypsinized epidermal suspension transplant works on the principle of regenerative medicine, and can be effectively utilized to treat post-traumatic scars. Radiofrequency ablation induces micro-injuries on to the scarred skin, PRP stimulates wound healing and the fat acts as a reservoir of adipocyte-derived stem cells while providing a cushioning effect. Furthermore, PRP may also promote regeneration of terminal nerve fibres.[33]

Method

- One-third of the size of the area to be treated was calculated and one-third the size of this area was selected as the donor site; this is usually on covered sites such as the upper lateral and anterior aspects of the thighs.

- The skin graft was immediately transferred to 0.25% trypsin–ethylenediaminetetraacetic acid solution in a petri dish. The petri dish was incubated at 40°C for 1.5 hours.
- In the meantime, PRP was prepared by drawing 10 ml of venous blood.
- The trypsinized skin graft was washed with platelet-poor plasma. The epidermis was teased out from the dermis with the help of a pair of blunt forceps; however, the tightly adherent dermis was left intact with the epidermal fragments. The glistening white dermis was discarded, and the brown epidermis was cut into tiny pieces and transferred to a test tube containing 1.5 ml of thick suspension of PRP.
- The cell suspension thus obtained contained dermo-epidermal fragments, containing cells from the basal cell layer including keratinocytes and melanocytes and parts of adherent dermis.
- This suspension was kept in the incubator at 37°C for one minute to make a homogenous cell suspension at body temperature.

Thus, a cocktail of radiofrequency ablation, PRP and skin fragments can be utilized for creating new skin, accelerating wound healing and reducing the need for tissue expanders or grafting.
The author has utilized this in various indications for augmenting post-procedure healing. (Figures 4a, 4b.)

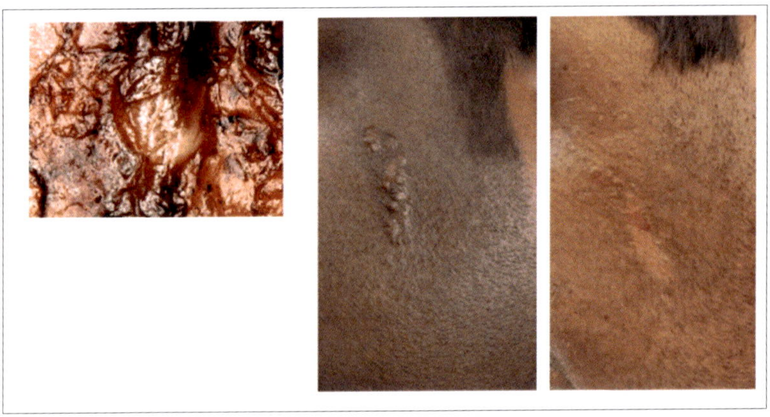

Figure 4a. Foreign body granuloma – Radiofrequency ablation with PRP-enriched epidermal suspension transplant after four weeks of procedure (RA-PEEST). The dermoscopic picture on the left shows a chalky white foreign body globule, the central one is baseline picture and last one 4 weeks after the procedure. Photo: Dr Suruchi Garg, Aura Skin Institute, Chandigarh, India.

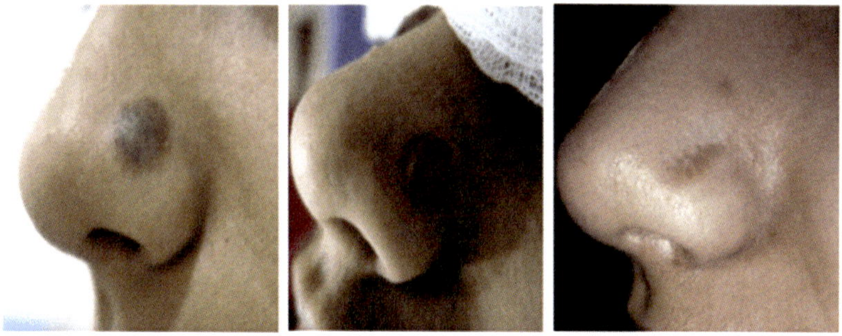

Figure 4b. Melanocytic nevus removal with radiofrequency ablation and PRP-enriched epidermal suspension transplant (RA-PEEST): baseline, two weeks, three months. Photo: Dr Suruchi Garg, Aura Skin Institute, Chandigarh, India.

Vitiligo

Autoreactive CD8+ T-cells are the primary suspect considered to be responsible for the destruction of melanocytes. Therefore, topical use of autoimmune inhibitors including those derived from MSCs, thanks to their immune-modulatory properties, have been reported to be successful in the promotion of re-pigmentation. MSCs can suppress the proliferation of CD8+ T via the NKG2D pathway while inducing T-cell apoptosis. The use of pharmacological agents for reducing cellular oxidative stress with the help of topical application of antioxidants and growth factors has also been in use. Intravenous administration of MSCs has been shown to regulate the level of reactive oxidative species (ROS) in a mice model. Growth factors derived from platelet-rich plasma (PRP) or from MSCs caused rapid tissue regeneration.

Finally, MSC therapy also has been shown to stimulate the mobilization of healthy melanocytes, leading to successful re-pigmentation of skin lesions in vitiligo patients.[40]

Cocktail of live cells and PRP in vitiligo surgery

Mechanism of action

PRP has a high concentration of GFs, particularly basic FGF (bFGF) and stem cell factors (SCF), which may stimulate melanocyte proliferation and re-pigmentation in the vitiligo lesions.[40,41] In addition, PRP enhances cellular proliferation, connective tissue healing, angiogenesis and collagen synthesis, resulting in faster graft uptake, improved chances of survival and reduced risk of infection.[42] PRP enhances hair melanocyte reserves and may reverse leukotrichia. It contains natural trypsin inhibitors and increases the viscosity of the suspension, thus preventing its runoff. This results in better melanocyte proliferation, survival and faster re-pigmentation.[42]

Technique

Recently, the authors proposed a new modified procedure as an effort to improve the outcome of vitiligo surgery using PRP as a suspending agent and erbium: yttrium aluminium garnet (Er: YAG) laser for ablating the recipient site, known as laser ablation on the recipient area with PRP-enriched epidermal suspension transplant (LA-PEEST) among 10 patients with vitiligo.

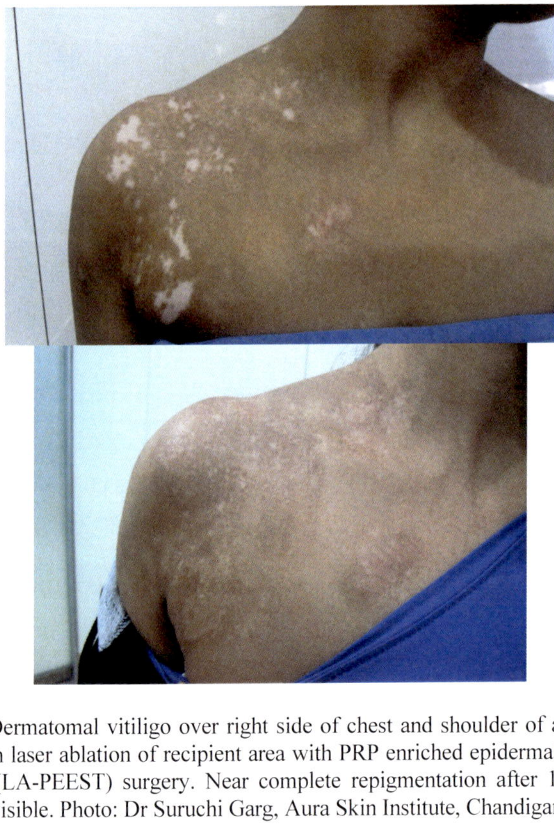

Figure 5. Dermatomal vitiligo over right side of chest and shoulder of a young girl treated with laser ablation of recipient area with PRP enriched epidermal suspension transplant (LA-PEEST) surgery. Near complete repigmentation after 12 weeks of surgery is visible. Photo: Dr Suruchi Garg, Aura Skin Institute, Chandigarh, India.

The epidermal stem cell suspension was prepared by the method described above under the section on wound healing. The achromic epidermis was removed by the Er: YAG laser with a conventional 2 mm spot-size tip at a fluence of 2,500 mJ/pass. A total of five passes were given at one area until pinpoint bleeds were appreciated on scrubbing with saline-dipped gauze, signifying ablation up to the dermo-epidermal junction. The suspension was poured evenly over the ablated surface; the tiny dermo-epidermal fragments were spread over the recipient area ensuring that the margins were covered evenly.[42] Re-pigmentation was observed as early as two weeks after the treatment. Of 20 lesions, 12 (60%) showed excellent response, of which 10 lesions (50%) showed complete re-pigmentation in eight weeks only. This study indicates that PRP-enriched epidermal suspension transplant (LA-PEEST) has the potential to improve the rate of healing and re-pigmentation in vitiligo patches.

Ageing

Stem cells have been marketed as a promising treatment for cutaneous rejuvenation due to their potential for self-renewal and differentiation, alone or as an adjuvant to microneedling or laser therapy.

Biophysical analysis has demonstrated increased elasticity and skin hydration in addition to decreased transepidermal water loss, roughness and melanin index, and increased dermal collagen and elastin on histopathology. However, more clinical data are needed to fully evaluate their effects and to develop standardized protocols.[43,44]

Between PRP and stem cells for anti-ageing, PPR has stronger evidence behind its use, especially when combined with other treatment modalities, including microneedling or laser therapy. PRP has been reported to improve dermal elasticity and skin texture via the stimulation of dermal fibro-enhancing the expression of matrix metalloproteinases (MMP) 1 and 3. Furthermore, it accelerates hyaluronic acid production and leads to improvement in skin hydration and volume, and various methods have been employed for the application of PRP in this indication including intradermal or topical PRP alone, or in combination with microneedling.[45,46]

Conclusion

The availability of sufficient studies investigating the use of human stem cells for cutaneous and aesthetic purposes is currently lacking. Early studies have begun to demonstrate promise regarding the efficacy of stem cells in various dermatological indications, especially when combined with other treatment modalities.

Furthermore, our understanding of their short- and long-term effects on safety remain limited and a complete understanding of their cellular and molecular interactions is lacking. Our current knowledge regarding their effect on neoplastic cells and tumorigenesis remains imprecise. Moreover, their isolation and processing is difficult and expensive, and these practical considerations limit their wide-scale use.

Large-scale clinical studies are warranted to fully understand their potential and to develop standardized protocols.

In the present scenario, it seems prudent to utilize PRP along with epidermal cell suspension as a cocktail of live cells, which augments the regenerative and regrowth potential of the former, for longer-lasting results with more sustained effect. Follicular suspension is yet another easily accessible and promising new modality in the field of vitiligo surgery, patterned hair loss and alopecia areata, which warrants detailed, in-depth studies in the future.

References

1. Garg S. Research article use of stem cells in intervention dermatology and trichology: a new hope. *SRDT*. 2019 Apr 10;**5**:1-8.
2. Herzog EL, Chai L, Krause DS. Plasticity of marrow-derived stem cells. *Blood* 2003;**102**:3483-93.
3. Schofield R. The relationship between the spleen colony-forming cell and the haemopoietic stem cell. *Blood Cells* 1978;**4**:7-25.
4. Monti M, Perotti C, Del Fante C, Cervio M, Redi CA. Stem cells: sources and therapies. *Biol Res*. 2012;**45**:207-14.
5. Prodinger CM, Reichelt J, Bauer JW, Laimer M. Current and future perspectives of stem cell therapy in dermatology. *Ann Dermatol*. 2017;**29**:667-87.
6. Ulloa-Montoya F, Verfaillie CM, Hu WS. Culture systems for pluripotent stem cells. *J Biosci Bioeng* 2005;**100**:12-27.
7. Khandpur S, Gupta S, Gunaabalaji DR. Stem cell therapy in dermatology. *IJDVL*. 2021 Jun 24;**87**:753-67.
8. Verfaillie C. Pluripotent stem cells. *Transfusion Clinique et Biologique*. 2009 May 1;**16**:65-e9.
9. Novus Biologicals. Mesenchymal stem cells. Abingdon, UK: Novus Biologicals [no updated date; cited 21 Mar 2022] [Internet]. Available from:

https://www.novusbio.com/research-areas/stem-cells/mesenchymal-stem-cell-markers
10. Asakawa K, Toyoshima KE, Ishibashi N, Tobe H, Iwadate A, Kanayama T, et al. Hair organ regeneration via the bioengineered hair follicular unit transplantation. *Sci Rep*. 2012;**2**:424.
11. Balañá ME, Charreau HE, Leirós GJ. Epidermal stem cells and skin tissue engineering in hair follicle regeneration. *World J Stem Cells*. 2015;**7**:711-727.
12. Gentile P, Scioli MG, Bielli A, Orlandi A, Cervelli V. Stem cells from human hair follicles: first mechanical isolation for immediate autologous clinical use in androgenetic alopecia and hair loss. *Stem Cell Investig*. 2017;**4**:58.
13. Teumer J, Cooley J. Follicular cell implantation: an emerging cell therapy for hair loss. *Semin Plast Surg*. 2005;**19**:193-200.
14. Gentile P, Garcovich S. Advances in regenerative stem cell therapy in androgenic alopecia and hair loss: Wnt pathway, growth-factor, and mesenchymal stem cell signaling impact analysis on cell growth and hair follicle development. *Cells*. 2019;**8**:E466.
15. Gentile P, Cole JP, Cole MA, Garcovich S, Bielli A, Scioli MG, et al. Evaluation of not-activated and activated PRP in hair loss treatment: role of growth factor and cytokine concentrations obtained by different collection systems. *Int J Mol Sci*. 2017;**18**:E408.
16. Hamed Kadry M, Kheir WAE, Sayed Shalaby ME, El Shahid AR, Metwally HG. Autologous adipose derived stem cell versus platelet rich plasma injection in the treatment of androgentic alopecia: efficacy, side effects and safety. *J Clin Exp Dermatol Res* 2018;**9**:1000447 [no updated date; cited 27 March 2022] [Internet]. Available from: https://doi.org/10.4172/2155-9554.1000447.
17. Tak YJ, Lee SY, Cho AR, Kim YS. A randomized, double-blind, vehicle-controlled clinical study of hair regeneration using adipose-derived stem cell constituent extract in androgenetic alopecia. *Stem Cells Transl Med*. 2020 Aug 1;**9**:839-49.
18. Elmaadawi IH, Mohamed BM, Ibrahim ZAS, Abdou SM, El Attar YA, Youssef A, et al. Stem cell therapy as a novel therapeutic intervention for resistant cases of alopecia areata and androgenetic alopecia. *J Dermatolog Treat*. 2018 Jul 4;**29**:431-40.
19. Fawzy MM, Gabr HM, El Maadawi ZM. Autologous progenitor cell implantation as a novel therapeutic intervention for alopecia areata. *J Egypt Women's Dermatologic Soc*. 2011 Jan;**8**:11-6.

20. Anderi R, Makdissy N, Azar A, Rizk F, Hamade A. Cellular therapy with human autologous adipose-derived adult cells of stromal vascular fraction for alopecia areata. *Stem Cell Res Ther*. 2018 May 15;**9**:141.
21. Eremia S, Newman N. Long-term follow-up after autologous fat grafting: analysis of results from 116 patients followed at least 12 months after receiving the last of a minimum of two treatments. *Dermatol Surg*. 2000 Dec;**26**:1150-8.
22. Kosaric N, Kiwanuka H, Gurtner GC. Stem cell therapies for wound healing. *Expert Opin Bio Ther*. 2019 Jun 3;**19**:575-85.
23. Agren MS, Steenfos HH, Dabelsteen S, Hansen JB, Dabelsteen E. Proliferation and mitogenic response to PDGF-BB of fibroblasts isolated from chronic venous leg ulcers is ulcer-age dependent. *J Invest Dermatol.* 1999 Apr;**112**:463-9.
24. Guenou H, Nissan X, Larcher F, Feteira J, Lemaitre G, Saidani M, et al. Human embryonic stem-cell derivatives for full reconstruction of the pluristratified epidermis: a preclinical study. *Lancet.* 2009 Nov 21;**374**:1745-53.
25. de Miguel-Beriain I. The ethics of stem cells revisited. *Adv Drug Deliv Rev.* 2015 Mar;82-83:176-80.
26. Wu YJ, Chen L, Scott PG, Tredget EE. Mesenchymal stem cells enhance wound healing through differentiation and angiogenesis. *Stem Cells*. 2007;**25**:2648-2659.
27. Liu L, Yu Y, Hou Y, Chai J, Duan H, Chu W, et al. Human umbilical cord mesenchymal stem cells transplantation promotes cutaneous wound healing of severe burned rats. *PLoS One*. 2014;**9**:e88348.
28. Zuk PA, Zhu M, Ashjian P, De Ugarte DA, Huang JI, Mizuno H, et al. Human adipose tissue is a source of multipotent stem cells. *Mol Biol Cell.* 2002 Dec;**13**:4279-95.
29. Garg RK, Rennert RC, Duscher D, Sorkin M, Kosaraju R, Auerbach LJ, et al. Capillary force seeding of hydrogels for adipose-derived stem cell delivery in wounds. *Stem Cell Transl Med.* 2014 Sep;**3**:1079-1089.
30. Liao Y, Itoh M, Yang A, Zhu H, Roberts S, Highet AM, et al. Human cord blood-derived unrestricted somatic stem cells promote wound healing and have therapeutic potential for patients with recessive dystrophic epidermolysis bullosa. *Cell Transplant*. 2014 Mar;**23**:303-17.
31. Aguado BA, Mulyasasmita W, Su J, Lampe, KJ, Heilshorn SC. Improving viability of stem cells during syringe needle flow through the design of hydrogel cell carriers. *Tissue Eng Part A*. 2012 Apr;**18**:806-15.

32. Falanga V, Iwamoto S, Chartier M, Yufit T, Butmarc J, Kouttab N, et al. Autologous bone marrow-derived cultured mesenchymal stem cells delivered in a fibrin spray accelerate healing in murine and human cutaneous wounds. *J Invest Dermatol*. 2007 Apr;**127**:S49-S49.
33. Lee YS, Lim KS, Oh JE, Yoon A-R, Joo WS, Kim HS, et al. Development of porous PLGA/PEI1.8k biodegradable microspheres for the delivery of mesenchymal stem cells (MSCs). *J Control Release*. 2015 May 10;**205**:128-133.
34. Guo RJ, Ward CL, Davidson JM, Duvall CL, Wenke JC, Guelcher SA. A transient cell-shielding method for viable MSC delivery within hydrophobic scaffolds polymerized in situ. *Biomaterials*. 2015 Jun;**54**:21-33.
35. Rustad KC, Wong VW, Sorkin M, Glotzbach JP, Major MR, Rajadas J, et al. Enhancement of mesenchymal stem cell angiogenic capacity and stemness by a biomimetic hydrogel scaffold. *Biomaterials*. 2012 Jan;**33**:80-90.
36. Hare JM, Traverse JH, Henry TD, Dib N, Strumpf RK, Schulman SP, et al. A randomized, double-blind, placebo-controlled, dose-escalation study of intravenous adult human mesenchymal stem cells (prochymal) after acute myocardial infarction. *J American Col Cardiol*. 2009 Dec 8;**54**:2277-86.
37. Park JS, Suryaprakash S, Lao Y-H, Leong KW. Engineering mesenchymal stem cells for regenerative medicine and drug delivery. *Methods*. 2015 Aug;**84**:3-16.
38. Brandl A, Meyer M, Bechmann V, Nerlich M, Angele P. Oxidative stress induces senescence in human mesenchymal stem cells. *Exp Cell Res*. 2011 Jul 1;**317**:1541-1547.
39. Zahorec P, Sarkozyova N, Ferancikova N, Bukovcan P, Danisovic L, Bohac M, et al. Autologous mesenchymal stem cells application in post-burn scars treatment: a preliminary study. *Cell Tissue Bank*. 2021 Mar;**22**:39-46.
40. Parambath N, Sharma VK, Parihar AS, Sahni K, Gupta S. Use of platelet-rich plasma to suspend noncultured epidermal cell suspension improves repigmentation after autologous transplantation in stable vitiligo: a double-blind randomized controlled trial. *Int J Dermatol* 2019;**58**:472-6.
41. Kadry M, Tawfik A, Abdallah N, Badawi A, Shokeir H. Platelet-rich plasma versus combined fractional carbon dioxide laser with platelet-rich plasma in the treatment of vitiligo: a comparative study. *Clin Cosmet Investig Dermatol*. 2018;**11**:551-9.

42. Garg S, Dosapaty N, Arora AK. Laser ablation of the recipient area with platelet-rich plasma-enriched epidermal suspension transplant in vitiligo surgery: a pilot study. *Dermatol Surg*. 2019 Jan;**45**:83-9.
43. Wang JV, Schoenberg E, Saedi N, Ibrahim O. Platelet-rich plasma, collagen peptides, and stem cells for cutaneous rejuvenation. *J Clin Aesthet Dermatol*. 2020;**13**:44-49.
44. Zhou BR, Zhang T, Bin Jameel AA, Xu Yang, Xu Yan, Guo S-L, et al. The efficacy of conditioned media of adipose-derived stem cells combined with ablative carbon dioxide fractional resurfacing for atrophic acne scars and skin rejuvenation. *J Cosmet Laser Ther*. 2016;**18**:138-148.
45. Peng GL. Platelet-rich plasma for skin rejuvenation: facts, fiction, and pearls for practice. *Facial Plast Surg Clin North Am*. 2019 Aug;**27**:405-11.
46. Hesseler MJ, Shyam N. Platelet-rich plasma and its utility in the treatment of acne scars: a systematic review. *J Am Acad Dermatol*. 2019 Jun;**80**:1730-45.